A–Z of Orthopaedic Radiology

Commissioning Editor: Michael J. Houston
Project Editor: Sheila Black
Project Manager: Nora Naughton
Designer: Sarah Russell

A–Z of Orthopaedic Radiology

Sarah Burnett MBBS MRCP FRCR
Consultant Musculoskeletal Radiologist
St Mary's Hospital
London, UK

Andrew Taylor BSc MBBS FRCS
Specialist Registrar in Orthopaedics
Wexham Park Hospital
Slough, UK

Martin Watson MBBS FRCS FRCR
Specialist Registrar in Radiology
St Mary's Hospital
London, UK

W.B. SAUNDERS

London • Edinburgh • New York • Philadelphia • St Louis • Sydney • Toronto 2000

W. B. SAUNDERS
An imprint of Harcourt Publishers Limited

First published 2000

ISBN 0 7020 2492 9

British Library Cataloguing in Publication Data
A catalogue record for this book is available from the British Library

Library of Congress Cataloging in Publication Data
A catalog record for this book is available from the Library of Congress

Note
Medical knowledge is constantly changing. As new information becomes available, changes in treatment, procedures, equipment and the use of drugs become necessary. The editors/authors/contributors and the publishers have, as far as it is possible, taken care to ensure that the information given in this text is accurate and up to date. However, readers are strongly advised to confirm that the information, especially with regard to drug usage, complies with the latest legislation and standards of practice.

The
publisher's
policy is to use
**paper manufactured
from sustainable forests**

Printed in China

Contents

Glossary of terms and abbreviations

AAFB Acid-Alcohol Fast Bacillus

ABC Aneurysmal Bone Cyst

ANA Antinuclear antibody

AVM Arteriovenous malformation

AVN Avascular Necrosis

CRP C-Reactive Protein

CSF Cerebrospinal fluid

CT Computed Tomographic Scan

CTA Computed Tomographic Arthrogram

CXR Chest X-ray

EMG Electromyography

Equinus Plantar orientation of the foot

ESR Erythrocyte Sedimentation Rate

GCT Giant Cell Tumour

Hot Spot An area of increased activity on an isotope bone scan indicating high bone turnover

HPT Hyperparathyroidism

HRCT High Resolution Computed Tomographic Scan

HRT Hormone Replacement Therapy

LCH Langerhans Cell Histiocytosis (Histiocytosis X)

Madelung Deformity Poor development at the wrist due to metaphyseal abnormality

MC Metacarpal

MCP Metacarpophalangeal

Monomelic Affecting one limb

Monostotic Affecting one bone

MFH Malignant Fibrous Histiocytoma

MRA Magnetic Resonance Arthrogram

MR/MRI Magnetic Resonance Image

MT Metatarsal

MTP Metatarsophalangeal

NAI Non-Accidental Injury

NF Neurofibromatosis

OCD Osteochondritis Dissecans

Overtubulation Thin, gracile long bones

PCL Posterior Cruciate Ligament

Planus Flat

Platyspondyly Flattened vertebral bodies

Polyostotic Affecting multiple bones

PTH Parathormone

Rhizomelic Shortening of the proximal part of the limb

SBC Simple Bone Cyst

SCFE Slipped Capital Femoral Epiphysis

SXR Skull X-ray

T1 Weighting MR sequence giving low signal for water

T2 Weighting MR sequence giving high signal for water

TB Tuberculosis

Undertubulation Short, thickened long bones

US Ultrasound

Valgus Pointing away from the midline

Varus Pointing towards the midline

Acknowledgements

Thank you to Veronika and Dirk at the Institute of Orthopaedics, without whom this book would not have been possible.

Thank you also to all our colleagues, in Radiology, Orthopaedics and Rheumatology, who have provided advice and information.

Finally, thank you to Lesley, Jo, Chris, Perry and Xanthe, who have supported us collectively through the elephantine gestation period of this book.

Preface

This book is intended to be of use to specialist registrars training in both orthopaedics and radiology as a simple guide to orthopaedic radiology. The book can be used either to look up the radiological features of a known condition or to give some guidance as to the possible diagnosis for a given imaging appearance. A comprehensive range of musculoskeletal diseases is covered but acute trauma is not included (with the exception of non-accidental injury). Some rarer conditions are included as a guide for exams. The complications of trauma that may present to the fracture clinic are included.

Each condition is illustrated with a classic example of the pathology, imaged by plain films where possible or the best modality to demonstrate each pathology. The prime characteristics of the condition are given, together with the most common clinical presentation. Basic radiological features are listed, with suggestions for further imaging and non-radiological investigations. A brief description of the management is provided. The ⚷ symbol denotes a key point about the condition and ⚠ a warning. The conditions are listed in alphabetical order for ease of reference.

SB
AT
MW
January 2000

Achilles tendon tear

Characteristics
- **Age range:** Adults
- **Gender:** M > F
- **Incidence:** Not uncommon
- **Pathology:** It is likely that most ruptures occur in degenerate tendons.

Clinical presentation While pushing off with force, the patient feels as if he has been struck just above the heel. The patient cannot stand on tiptoe and the foot does not flex on squeezing the calf. There is often a palpable or visible gap in the tendon. The differential diagnosis is of a partial tear or a tear of the soleus muscle.

Radiology
Description
- MRI demonstrates discontinuity in the normal dark signal of the tendon, with an area of inhomogeneous increased signal

- ☛ US shows the disrupted tendon fibres with low, or mixed, echogenicity material in the gap
- 🕭 The preserved plantaris may be seen as a thin, normal tendon
- A partial tear may be well demonstrated on US as a focal area of abnormality

Further imaging
- None

Non-radiological investigations
- None

Management Conservative treatment in an equinus plaster may be appropriate, particularly in partial tears. If the ends cannot be brought together by conservative means then operative repair is required. Soleus tears can be treated by physiotherapy and a heel raise.

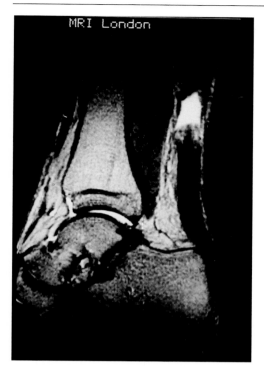

Fig 1.1 **T2-weighted sagittal MR of the ankle.**
There is discontinuity in the low signal of the
Achilles tendon with a focal high signal area
corresponding to the site of rupture.

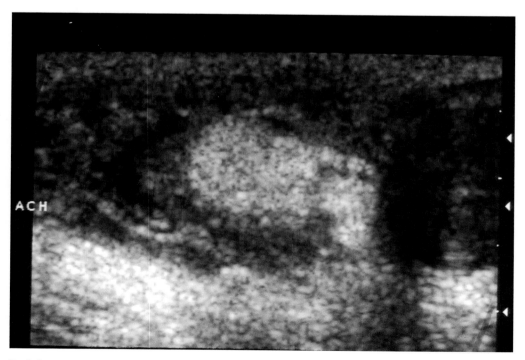

Fig 1.2 **Longitudinal US of the Achilles tendon.** The tendon has a gap in it filled with mixed
echogenicity material. The retracted distal end of tendon is seen on the right as it curls on itself.

2 Achondroplasia

Characteristics
- **Age range:** Presents from infancy to adulthood
- **Gender:** M = F
- **Incidence:** 1 in 10 000 – it is the commonest form of dwarfism
- **Pathology:** There is a hereditary defect of prebone cartilage causing reducing growth of cartilaginous bone. Membranous bone growth is unaffected.

Clinical presentation There is severe dwarfism with disproportionately short limbs, particularly the proximal parts (rhizomelia). There is macrocephaly, frontal bossing, a saddle nose, maxillary hypoplasia and prognathia. The lumbar lordosis is pronounced; there is progressive genu varum and short, broad hands with widening between the third and fourth fingers (trident hand). Intelligence and life expectancy are normal.

Radiology
Description
- ☞ Rhizomelic dwarfism, with disproportionately short ulnae and tibiae

- Large calvarium and frontal bossing
- Short ribs and a square inferior scapular margin
- Bullet-shaped vertebrae with posterior scalloping
- Increased height of vertebral interspace
- Narrow spinal canal and foramen magnum
- Upper lumbar angular kyphosis
- Short ilia and a narrow sacrum lead to a 'champagne-glass' pelvis
- Undertubulation of long bones
- Splayed bone ends with metaphyseal cupping
- Bowed limbs

Further imaging
- US/CT/MR may show hydrocephalus

Non-radiological investigations
- None

Management Human growth hormone may produce a short-term beneficial effect. Limb lengthening is successful. Narrowing of the foramen magnum and cervical or lumbar stenosis sometimes require decompression.

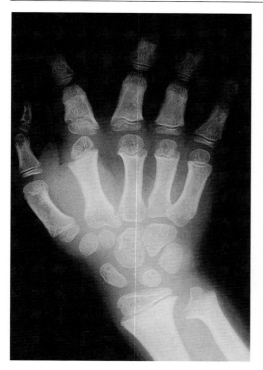

Fig 2.1 **DP hand.** The bones are markedly undertubulated and appear dense. There is a trident hand deformity.

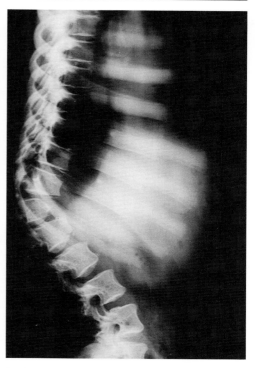

Fig 2.2 **Lateral spine.** There is central beaking of the vertebra at the level of the angular kyphosis.

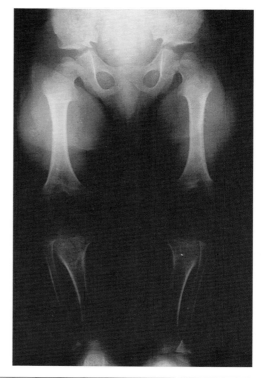

Fig 2.3 **AP both legs.** There is shortening of the limbs and splaying at the metaphyses. Short, square iliac wings and tight sciatic notches are demonstrated.

3 Acromegaly

Characteristics
- **Age range:** Adulthood. Excess growth hormone in children causes gigantism
- **Gender:** M = F
- **Incidence:** Rare
- **Pathology:** There is an excess of growth hormone from an anterior pituitary eosinophilic adenoma or hyperplasia. Excess hormone prior to epiphyseal fusion causes gigantism. After epiphyseal closure, only certain bones can respond to hormone, thus producing features of acromegaly.

Clinical presentation The classic features are of prognathism and enlargement of the lips, tongue and nose. The skin thickens, the thoracic cage enlarges and a kyphosis develops. The skull, hands and feet enlarge and the patient may complain that he needs to buy new hats, gloves and shoes! Diabetes, hypothyroidism, testicular atrophy and amenorrhoea are also associated.

Radiology
Description
- ☞ Heel pad thickness is increased
- Cartilage thickening leads to apparent joint space widening
- Vertebral bodies increase in height
- Pituitary fossa may be enlarged
- Mandibular hyperplasia
- Sites of muscle insertion become more prominent
- Premature arthritis is common

Further imaging
- CT or MR of the pituitary
- US of the abdomen to look for visceral enlargement

Non-radiological investigations
- Raised growth hormone levels which do not suppress with glucose
- Serum glucose and calcium are elevated

Management The underlying pituitary adenoma may require surgical resection.

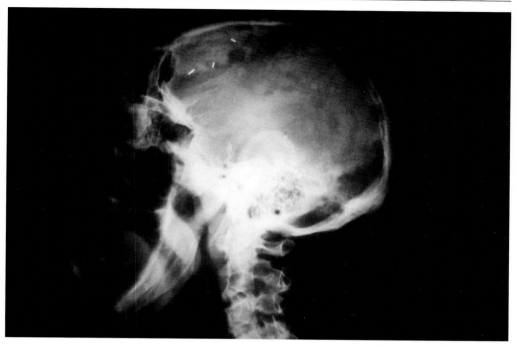

Fig 3.1 **Lateral skull.** Note the large frontal sinuses, prognathism and ballooned pituitary fossa.

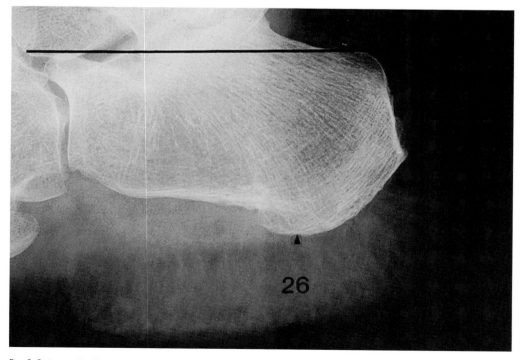

Fig 3.2 **Lateral calcaneum.** The heel pad thickness is increased.

4 Acute osteomyelitis

Characteristics
- **Age range:** Most commonly affects children aged 5–15 years
- **Gender:** M = F
- **Incidence:** Not uncommon
- **Pathology:** Bone infection may occur by haematogenous or direct spread. Bacteria enter the bone via the nutrient artery and multiply in the metaphysis where blood flow is slower through the sinusoids. There is an increased risk in patients with sickle cell disease and IV drug users. It occurs more frequently in the lower limb and 85% of cases are due to staphylococcus species. Increased pressure in affected bone leads to ischaemic necrosis and devascularized segments form sequestra.

Clinical presentation The onset of osteomyelitis is preceded by penetrating injury, sore throat, chest infection or urinary tract infection. There is fever, generalized malaise and localized pain. The affected bone is hot and tender to palpation and there is muscle spasm.

Radiology
Description
- ☀ Plain films may be normal for 7–10 days
- A periosteal reaction develops
- Permeative bone destruction is seen along the metadiaphysis
- Acute infection may appear very similar to Ewing's sarcoma

Further imaging
- Bone scan and MR are highly sensitive to the early changes
- MR may show high signal on T2 due to oedema or abscess formation
- US of a long bone may demonstrate a subperiosteal abscess, particularly in children, due to the loose periosteum
- Imaging-guided biopsy may be necessary to identify an organism

Non-radiological investigations
- Histology and MC+S
- Raised white count, positive blood cultures

Management Intravenous antibiotics should be given as soon as the diagnosis is suspected. A prolonged course may be required. Analgesia with or without splinting is given for symptomatic relief. If there is no response within 24 hours or there is a subperiosteal abscess then drainage may be required. Inadequate or delayed treatment can lead to chronic osteomyelitis.

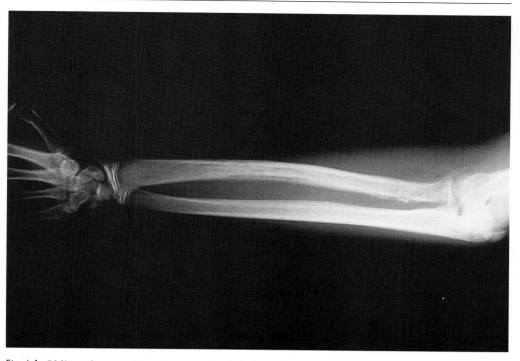

Fig 4.1 **Oblique forearm.** There is permeative lytic bone destruction and periosteal reaction.

5 Aneurysmal bone cyst

Characteristics
- **Age range:** Most common in the first and second decades; peak age 16 years
- **Gender:** Slight female preponderance
- **Incidence:** 10% of all benign bone tumours
- **Pathology:** The majority are primary, although some do occur secondary to other tumours such as GCT. The cyst contains clotted blood and microscopically shows fibrosis with large vascular spaces and multinucleated giant cells.

Clinical presentation
The rapidly expanding lesions characteristically cause pain with a visible or palpable mass.

Radiology
Description
- ☞ A highly expansile, metaphyseal, lytic lesion
- The cortex is markedly thinned but not usually breached
- Rapid growth is seen which may lead to a wide zone of transition

Further imaging
- CT or MR may show fluid–fluid levels from repeated haemorrhage
- Imaging-guided biopsy

Non-radiological investigations
- Histology

Management
Very rarely, lesions may undergo spontaneous regression. Curettage and bone grafting are performed, although the graft may resorb with recurrence of the cyst. Packing with methylmethacrylate may be more effective. For proximal humerus or femur, en bloc resection and endoprosthetic replacement may be necessary.

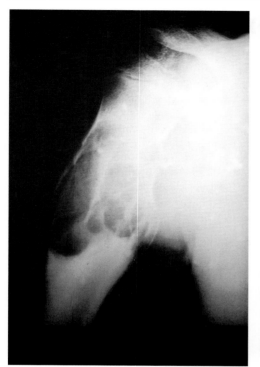

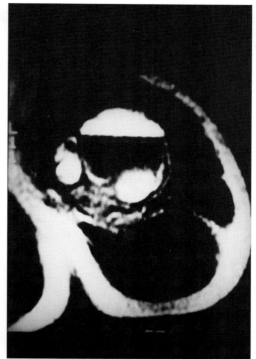

Fig 5.1 **AP shoulder.** There is a markedly
expansile multiloculate lytic lesion in the
metadiaphysis with a pathological fracture.

Fig 5.2 **T2-weighted coronal MR of femur.**
Fluid–fluid levels are noted within the lesion due
to layering of haemorrhage of different ages.

6 Ankylosing spondylitis

Characteristics
- **Age range:** Most often presents between the ages of 15 and 35 years
- **Gender:** M:F = at least 5:1
- **Incidence:** Three times more common in whites
- **Pathology:** There is a genetic predisposition associated with the HLA B27 antigen. There are probably also environmental triggers. It is associated with ulcerative colitis, iritis and aortic insufficiency; pulmonary fibrosis also occurs in 1%. Synovitis of the sacroiliac and costovertebral joints leads to destruction of cartilage and bone. Inflammation of the fibroosseous junctions affects intervertebral discs, ligaments and insertions of large tendons. Ossification of fibrous tissue leads to bony ankylosis and the typical spinal syndesmophytes.

Clinical presentation The patient suffers an insidious onset of low back pain and stiffness. Stiffness progresses along the spine which may become completely rigid; 10–20% of patients also have an inflammatory arthritis in a large joint.

Radiology
Description
- Changes start at the thoracolumbar junction
- Early erosions in the margins of the endplates are followed by healing changes, leading to the 'squared off' appearance of the vertebral bodies (Romanus lesion)
- ☞ Flowing syndesmophytes eventually result in a 'bamboo spine'
- Posterior elements may also fuse
- The sacroiliac joints demonstrate erosive changes followed by healing and obliteration of the joints

Further imaging
- Bone scanning may demonstrate increased uptake at the sacroiliac joints
- CT of the sacroiliac joints to look for erosions
- MR of the sacroiliac joints to look for oedema

Non-radiological investigations
- HLA B27 status
- Raised ESR and CRP during the acute phase

Management Analgesics and antiinflammatory agents are given for symptomatic relief. Physiotherapy may alleviate stiffness and maintain movement. Joint replacement may be required for peripheral joint disease. With severe cases spinal surgery may be indicated.

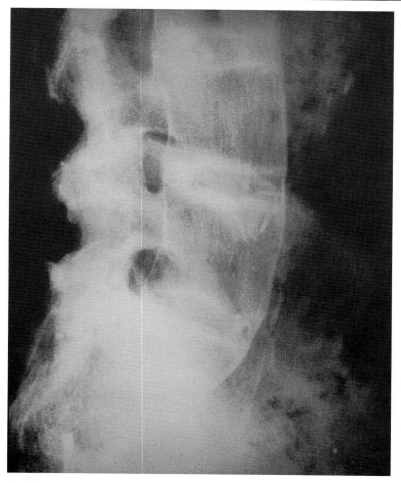

Fig 6.1 **Lateral spine.** There is bridging syndesmophyte formation across the vertebral bodies with squaring and sclerosis of the endplates. Note complete fusion of the posterior elements.

7 Anterior cruciate ligament (ACL) tear

Characteristics
- **Age range:** Generally young adults
- **Gender:** M > F (due to contact sports)
- **Incidence:** Common
- **Pathology:** The ACL consists of the anteromedial and larger posterolateral bands. Tears generally occur due to a combined rotation and impaction injury to the knee while weight bearing and flexed. Partial tears of the anteromedial band may occur. There is a high incidence of progression to complete tears. ACL tears do not heal.

Clinical presentation There is a history of early swelling following injury (within one hour). The patient is usually unable to continue with normal activities. The patient may hear a 'pop' or 'snap'. The anterior draw sign, Lachmann's and the pivot shift test are positive, although they are difficult and sometimes impossible to elicit in the acutely injured knee. Late presentation is with a feeling of instability and giving way. Patients may present with associated meniscal pathology such as pain and locking. Seventy percent of patients with traumatic haemarthroses will have sustained an ACL tear and 56% of knees with recent ACL tears have lateral meniscal tears. In patients presenting with chronic ACL deficient knees, medial meniscal tears are more common.

Radiology
Description
- Plain films may show an effusion at the time of the injury
- Rarely, a small avulsion fracture of the anterior tibial spine is identified

- ⚷ MR demonstrates abnormal or absent signal from the anterior cruciate ligament
- Anterior displacement of the tibia may be evident
- 🔔 There may be associated meniscal, osteochondral injury or bone bruising, particularly in the lateral compartment

Further imaging
- Osteochondral injury may require evaluation with MR arthrography to check the integrity of the overlying cartilage

Non-radiological investigations
- None

Management In the acute phase, the haemarthrosis can be aspirated and physiotherapy commenced to maintain range of movement and muscle strength. Non-operative management involves proprioceptive physiotherapy and bracing or orthotics. Surgery is indicated for symptomatic meniscal pathology and/or symptomatic instability and depends on age, preinjury level of activity, occupation and motivation. Surgery should not be performed in the acute phase and delayed until swelling, pain, inflammation and stiffness have resolved. The ligament can be reconstructed by open or arthroscopic methods, using the middle third of the patellar tendon or a four-strand hamstring graft. Extensive postoperative rehabilitation is necessary and patients can expect to return to full sporting activity 9 months after surgery. Degenerative change in the knee after injury is probably due to associated subchondral injury rather than long-term instability.

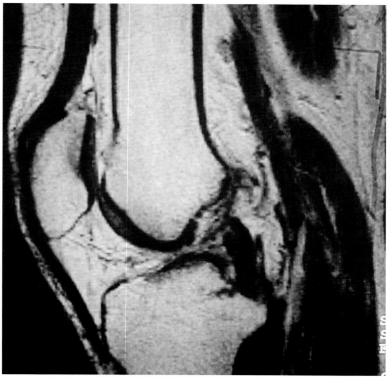

Fig 7.1 **T1-weighted sagittal MR of the knee.** There is virtually no normal signal from the anterior cruciate ligament.

8 Avascular necrosis (AVN)

Characteristics
- **Age range:** Commonly seen in the third to fifth decades
- **Gender:** M > F, especially in the idiopathic form
- **Incidence:** Not uncommon; bilateral in 50% (80% if secondary to steroids)
- **Pathology:** Twenty-five percent of cases have no predisposing cause. Others are due to impaired arterial supply secondary to trauma, e.g. fracture; occlusion, e.g. sickle cell disease; capillary compression, e.g. Gaucher's disease; or fatty infiltration, e.g. steroids. Leads to bone death.

Clinical presentation AVN most often affects the femoral head but can occur at the end of any long bone and in the spine, particularly in sickle cell disease. The earliest stages are asymptomatic and the patient may present some time after the blood supply has been disrupted; 75% will show progression within 3 years. Pain is the commonest complaint. The joint may later become stiff and deformed. If the bone is palpable then it may be tender.

Radiology
Description
- ☀ Initially plain films are normal
- Remaining 'live' bone becomes osteopenic
- Infarcted bone becomes sclerotic, with serpiginous lines
- Subchondral lucency develops parallel with the bone end
- Cortical collapse occurs

Further imaging
- ☞ MR is indicated before the plain films become abnormal. The appearances are variable depending on the stage of disease
- Alteration in marrow signal is seen. Eventually subchondral low-signal 'tramlines' develop

Non-radiological investigations
- Appropriate investigation of underlying pathology
- Intramedullary pressure is raised and can be measured with a metaphyseal cannula

Management There is no place for conservative treatment with protected weight bearing, as it does not alter the progression of destruction. Core decompression is useful in the early stages although 30% will still progress despite treatment. Cortical bone grafts have been used prior to collapse but the results are poor. The use of electrical stimulation by pulsed magnetic fields remains controversial. Realignment osteotomies can be used for localized areas of necrosis to transfer load to an undamaged part of the joint. Once necrosis is advanced with severe joint dysfunction, arthroplasty is indicated. Rarely, arthrodesis may be necessary.

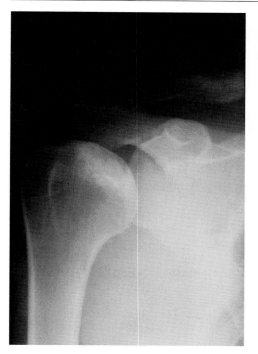

Fig 8.1 **AP shoulder.** There is sclerosis of the humeral head and a well-defined subchondral lucency.

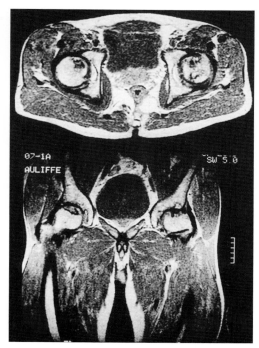

Fig 8.2 **Axial and coronal T1-weighted hip MR.** Note the low-signal serpiginous lines in the subchondral bone.

9 Baker's cyst

Characteristics
- **Age range:** Seen at any age
- **Gender:** M = F
- **Incidence:** Common
- **Pathology:** The lesion, also known as a popliteal cyst, is a synovial cyst at the back of the knee. It is formed by the escape of synovial fluid which is trapped by a one-way valve mechanism. This commonly occurs when the underlying joint is arthritic.

Clinical presentation Patients may present with pain or palpable mass. It may cause mechanical dysfunction and on occasion ruptures to cause a painful calf swelling, mimicking a DVT.

Radiology
Description
- Plain films may show a vague soft tissue mass behind the knee
- Associated degenerative changes may be seen
- US is the investigation of choice, demonstrating a 'speech bubble'-shaped, fluid-filled structure in the popliteal fossa, which communicates with the joint

Further imaging
- A Baker's cyst may be noted at MR

Non-radiological investigations
- None

Management It is possible to give symptomatic relief by aspiration of the cyst and steroid injection may delay recurrence. Baker's cyst may even recur following surgical excision as the underlying joint remains abnormal.

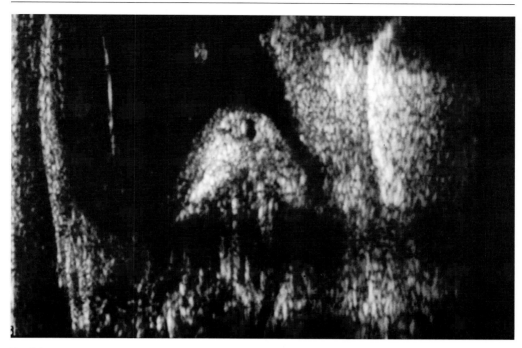

Fig 9.1 **Transverse US scan of the popliteal fossa.** A large fluid-filled structure can be seen, with a 'tongue' extending into the joint. It contains some internal echoes.

10 Blount's disease

Characteristics

- **Age range:** Most often toddlers, but there is a less common adolescent form
- **Gender:** M < F
- **Incidence:** Rare, but more common in African Americans, early walkers and obese toddlers
- **Pathology:** Affects the medial proximal tibial metaphysis. In spite of the historical name of osteochondrosis deformans, there is no histological evidence of avascular necrosis. Histology is similar to SUFE – acellular fibrosis, densely packed hypertrophic cartilage and transphyseal blood vessels. There is a genetic predisposition and ligamentous laxity may be an aetiological factor. The femoral epiphysis may also be affected.

Clinical presentation Progressive bow-leg deformity usually associated with internal rotation of the tibia; 60% are bilateral. The adolescent form is milder and often unilateral.

Radiology

Description

- 🔑 Irregularity of medial tibial metaphysis with a posteromedial beak-like projection
- Enlargement and deformity of the medial tibial condyle

Further imaging

- None

Non-radiological investigations

- None

Management If bracing is started under the age of 3 there is 50–80% success. Osteotomy is indicated if a neutral tibio-femoral axis is not achieved after 1 year of treatment or in children over 4 years of age.

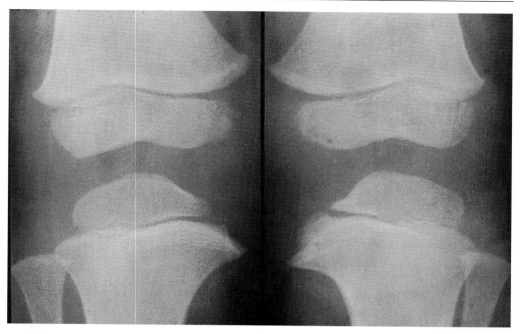

Fig 10.1 **AP both knees.** There is abnormal modelling and some new bone formation at the medial proximal tibial metaphysis in the left knee.

11 Bone bruise

Characteristics
- **Age range:** Most often seen in young adults
- **Gender:** M > F
- **Incidence:** Common
- **Pathology:** Acute trauma causes microfractures in the subchondral bone which may or may not be associated with cortical impaction.

Clinical presentation The patient may have pain following an injury unaccounted for by findings at arthroscopy.

Radiology
Description
- Appearances depend on the age of the lesion
- ☞ MR demonstrates high signal in the subchondral bone on T2 and fat-suppressed sequences in the acute lesion, while on T1 sequences signal is reduced due to oedema
- 🔔 On T2-weighted images alone, the signal may appear the same as that of the surrounding bone marrow
- As the bone bruise heals and becomes sclerotic, loss of signal is seen on all sequences
- There may be associated cortical impaction and chondral damage

Further imaging
- MRA to assess the cartilage over the defect

Non-radiological investigations
- None

Management Pain usually resolves in time but, depending on the severity of the injury, premature osteoarthritis may develop.

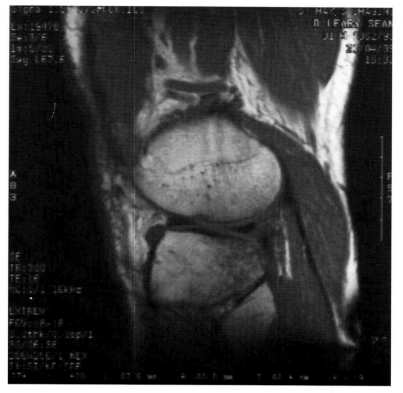

Fig 11.1 **T1-weighted sagittal MR of the knee.** There is impaction of the cortical surface with loss of signal, indicating local oedema. The overlying cartilage is probably intact.

12 Bone infarct

Characteristics

- **Age range:** May present at any age, depending on the aetiology
- **Gender:** M = F
- **Incidence:** Uncommon
- **Pathology:** May be medullary or cortical due to compression of nutrient artery and periosteal vessels. Can be secondary to conditions causing vascular compromise (such as sickle cell disease, excess steroids, trauma or inflammation) or idiopathic. It may be complicated by growth disturbance, early degenerative change or malignancy, malignant fibrous histiocytoma being the most common.

Clinical presentation Acute infarction may be painful but many cases are incidental findings. Increasing pain in a patient with a known infarct may be due to malignant change.

Radiology

Description
- ☞ Serpiginous dense lines are seen in the metadiaphysis

- May be single site or multiple, depending on the underlying pathology
- 🔔 Superimposed permeative destructive changes may be due to malignant change

Further imaging

- MR demonstrates 'tramlines' of low signal on all sequences in the mature infarct
- Malignant change is identified by a mass and high signal on T2-weighted sequences
- Imaging-guided biopsy may be appropriate

Non-radiological investigations

- Appropriate to investigating the underlying cause
- Histology for malignant change

Management Treatment of the underlying cause. Growth arrest, degenerative change or malignancy may require surgical treatment.

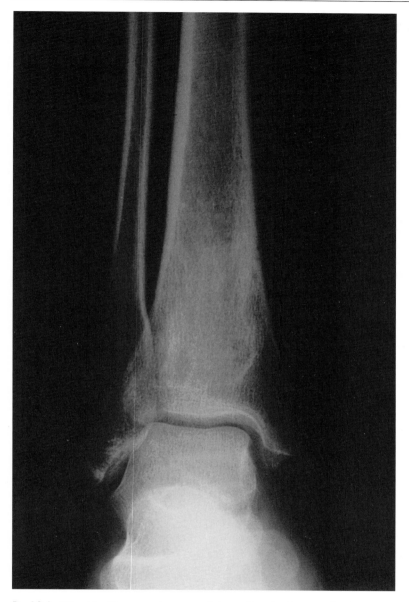

Fig 12.1 **AP ankle.** There are dense, serpiginous lines in the metaphysis.

13 Bone island

Characteristics
- **Age range:** Any age
- **Gender:** M = F
- **Incidence:** Very common
- **Pathology:** A nest of compact lamellar bone with an interspersed Haversian system. It is possibly a hamartoma or an error of endochondral ossification which fails to undergo remodelling. Forty percent may demonstrate slow growth, particularly in the growing skeleton. Some eventually disappear.

Clinical presentation An incidental finding.

Radiology
Description
- Solitary small (2 mm–2 cm) area of dense bone
- ☞ Well-circumscribed area of sclerosis with thorny radiations producing a 'brush border'
- Most common in pelvis, upper femora and spine

Further imaging
- May show activity on bone scan in the growing skeleton

Non-radiological investigations
- None

Management None, but may require differentiation from an osteoid osteoma or a sclerotic metastasis.

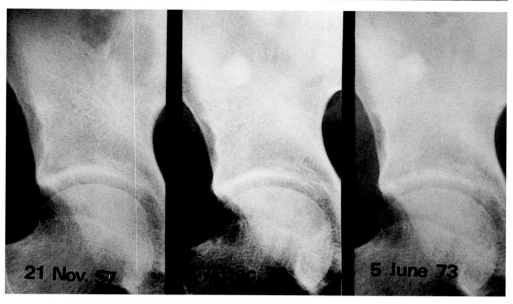

Fig 13.1 **AP hip.** This series of films demonstrates the gradual appearance of a bone island in the maturing skeleton. It is a small, dense, well-defined lesion.

14 Cavernous haemangioma

Characteristics
- **Age range:** Most common in the fourth to fifth decades
- **Gender:** M:F = 1:2
- **Incidence:** Up to 10% in some series
- **Pathology:** The lesions are hamartomas or arteriovenous malformations.

Clinical presentation May be an incidental finding on lumbar plain films or, rarely, may present with pain due to collapse.

Radiology
Description
- ☞ Prominent vertical striations are seen in a vertebral body
- Most common in the thoracic and lumbar spine
- Multiple in up to 30%

Further imaging
- MR demonstrates lesions not seen on plain films, usually bright on both T1 and T2 weighting
- CT appearances of prominent trabeculae are also characteristic

Non-radiological investigations
- None

Management Treatment is rarely necessary and is largely supportive if there is pain or collapse of the vertebral body.

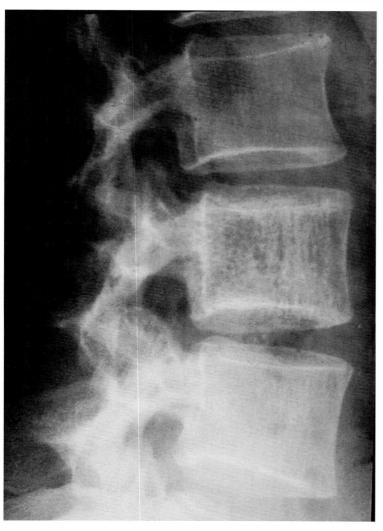

Fig 14.1 **Lateral spine.** Note the vertical striations in the affected vertebral body.

15 **Chondroblastoma**

Characteristics
- **Age range:** Most frequent in the second and third decades
- **Gender:** M > F
- **Incidence:** Rare
- **Pathology:** This is a benign tumour of immature cartilage cells. It is highly cellular with round or polygonal cells with eosinophilic cytoplasm. Scattered mitotic figures are not uncommon but malignant transformation does not occur. Giant cells are generally present.

Clinical presentation Patients generally present with a constant ache in the joint, usually the shoulder, knee or ankle. There may be bone tenderness next to the epiphysis.

Radiology
Description
- ☞ A well-defined lesion is seen in the epiphysis
- There is a small rim of reactive sclerosis
- 50% show calcification
- There may be extension into the metaphysis

Further imaging
- 🔔 MR, CT and bone scanning are all non-specific
- Imaging-guided biopsy

Non-radiological investigations
- Histology

Management The lesion is resected, generally after cessation of growth to avoid physeal damage. Curettage and cryosurgery are recommended although the local recurrence rate is 5–10%, which may eventually lead to joint replacement.

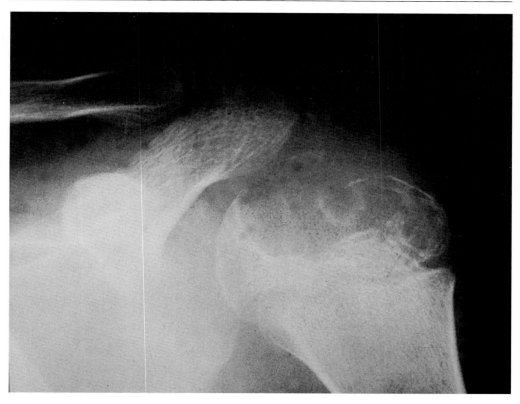

Fig 15.1 **AP shoulder.** There is a relatively well-defined, predominantly lytic lesion in the proximal humeral epiphysis. This does, however, show a degree of calcification within it.

16 **Chondrocalcinosis**

Characteristics

- **Age range:** Adult, generally over 60 years of age if idiopathic. When seen in younger patients, it is suggestive of a metabolic disorder or a familial form.
- **Gender:** M < F
- **Incidence:** Very common
- **Pathology:** There is calcium pyrophosphate dihydrate deposition in cartilage. It is seen in hyperparathyroidism, haemochromatosis, pseudogout and osteoarthritis. Rarely, it may be familial. Deposits occur both in hyaline and articular cartilage and in fibrocartilage.

Clinical presentation Usually the condition is asymptomatic but it may present with features of the underlying cause. In particular, pseudogout is characterized by attacks of acute arthritis.

Radiology

Description

- ⚷ Fine lines of calcium are identified running parallel to the joint surfaces or triangular-shaped densities in cartilage
- Most commonly seen in the knees and wrists

Further imaging

- None

Non-radiological investigations

- Serum calcium
- Analysis of joint effusions

Management Treat the underlying cause. Chondrocalcinosis, in itself, does not require treatment.

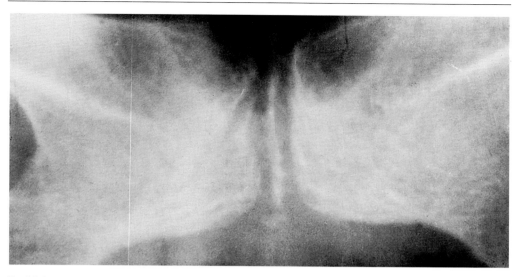

Fig 16.1 **AP pubic symphysis.** There is a dense band of calcification in the symphyseal cartilage.

17 Chondromyxoid fibroma

Characteristics

- **Age range:** Presents usually in the second and third decades
- **Gender:** Slight male preponderance
- **Incidence:** Rare
- **Pathology:** The tumour contains mucinous material and is partly cartilaginous. Malignant change is extremely rare.

Clinical presentation It may present as an incidental finding on radiography or as a pathological fracture, usually occurring in the lower limb.

Radiology

Description

- ⚷ A well-defined lytic lesion with residual trabeculae is seen, commonly in the anterior tibia
- Very rarely, matrix mineralization may occur

Further imaging

- Imaging-guided biopsy
- MR may define the local anatomy further

Non-radiological investigations

- Histology

Management The lesion generally should be excised but often it is only possible to perform bone graft and curettage. There is a high rate of recurrence.

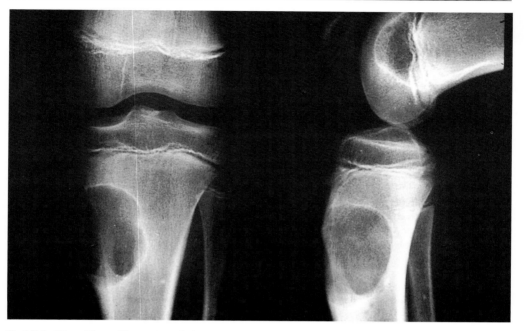

Fig 17.1 **AP and lateral knee.** A well-defined lucency is noted in the proximal tibial metaphysis.

18 Chondrosarcoma

Characteristics
- **Age range:** Most commonly seen in the fourth, fifth and sixth decades
- **Gender:** M:F = 1.5:1
- **Incidence:** The third most common primary bone tumour
- **Pathology:** May arise in preexisting benign cartilaginous tumours, 1% of which undergo malignant transformation. Thus it is more common in conditions such as Ollier's or Mafucci's syndrome (see p. 132). The basic neoplastic tissue is cartilage without evidence of direct osteoid formation, although bone may form from differentiation of cartilage. There are five types, most commonly central or peripheral (76%), though it can be mesenchymal, dedifferentiated or clear cell. Central form within a bone and peripheral from the surface of a bone.

Clinical presentation Peripheral tumours may enlarge without pain and local symptoms only develop because of mechanical irritation. Central tumours present with dull pain and a mass is rarely present. Common sites are the pelvis, femur and shoulder girdle.

Radiology
Description
- ☞ An aggressive, lytic lesion with 'chondroid' calcification
- Wide zone of transition
- Cortical destruction with a soft tissue mass
- Slow-growing lesions show cortical thickening
- Very slow-growing lesions may be indistinguishable from enchondroma
- 🔔 In a preexisting osteochondroma, malignant change may be indicated by rapid enlargement of the cartilage cap and destruction of existing benign calcification

Further imaging
- Imaging-guided biopsy
- MR for local staging
- Chest CT and bone scan for distant staging

Non-radiological investigations
- Histology

Management The tumour tends to be slow growing and metastasize late; therefore it is treated by wide excision and possibly prosthetic replacement. Generally chondrosarcoma is not chemo- or radiosensitive but adjuvant chemotherapy is considered in high-grade lesions and radical radiotherapy is useful for local control in unresectable or inoperable tumours.

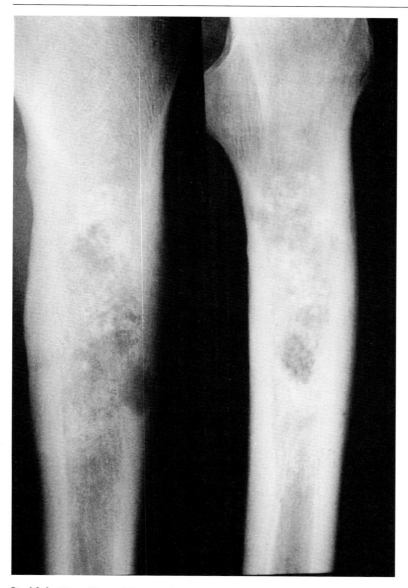

Fig 18.1 **AP and lateral femur.** There is an ill-defined area of a mixture of bony destruction and chondroid new bone formation. A more destructive area can be identified in the cortex.

19 Chronic granulomatous disease

Characteristics
- **Age range:** Children
- **Gender:** M >> F
- **Incidence:** Rare
- **Pathology:** It is more commonly an X-linked disorder affecting males but some females are affected by autosomal recessive transmission. The granulomatous response results from an inability of leucocytes to kill certain organisms after phagocytosis. This happens in the skeleton and other organs.

Clinical presentation There are chronic and recurrent suppurative infections. Patients may present with pain in the affected bones or unexplained fever. Dermatitis is often seen.

Radiology
Description
- ☞ Multiple metaphyses may be affected, often in a symmetrical distribution
- Destructive lesions or, more commonly, diffuse sclerosis may be seen

- In long-standing disease the entire bone may become affected and there is often modelling deformity
- Hilar adenopathy and eventual honeycomb lung

Further imaging
- Bone scanning demonstrates the multiplicity of the lesions
- CT or MR may further characterize the bony architecture
- Imaging-guided biopsy may be appropriate
- Visceral infections may require imaging

Non-radiological investigations
- ESR and CRP may be raised
- MC+S or histology may be of use in identifying organisms

Management Depends on the severity of the disease. Infections are treated as necessary.

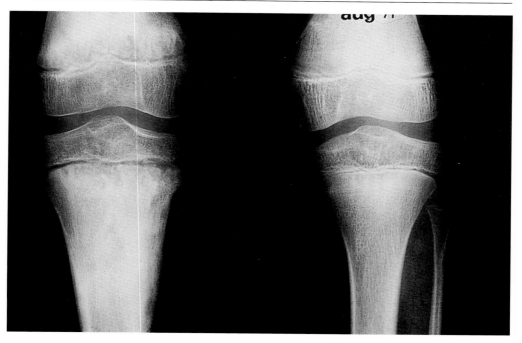

Fig 19.1 **AP both knees.** There is increased density and modelling deformity in the distal femoral and proximal tibial metaphyses.

20 Chronic osteomyelitis

Characteristics
- **Age range:** May occur at any age but more common in children as a consequence of acute osteomyelitis.
- **Gender:** M = F
- **Incidence:** Uncommon
- **Pathology:** May follow acute osteomyelitis, an open fracture or surgery. Devitalized bone occurs at the site of infection and cavities containing pus and necrotic bone (sequestra) develop. These are surrounded by relatively vascular bone and reactive new bone formation. Sinuses may form to the skin. The usual infecting organisms are *Staph. aureus, E. coli, Strep. pyogenes, proteus* and *pseudomonas* species. There may be fungal or tuberculous infection. If there is a prosthesis then *Staph. epidermidis* is the most common agent.

Clinical presentation There is often a chronic discharging sinus with thickened tissue and excoriation of the surrounding skin. It may present with an acute 'flare' – pain, pyrexia, redness and a purulent discharge from the sinus. Squamous carcinoma may develop in skin adjacent to the sinus in approximately 0.5% of patients. Pathological fractures occur.

Radiology
Description
- A lytic area is surrounded by a sclerotic rim of varying size
- Predominant sclerosis with little lysis may be seen
- A piece of dead bone may remain within the abscess cavity – the sequestrum

- In the metaphysis, the lesion may be more rounded and is termed a Brodie's abscess
- Long-standing infection can lead to periosteal reaction and modelling deformity

Further imaging
- MR or CT may further characterize the bony abnormality
- CT or fluoroscopy may be used to guide biopsy

Non-radiological investigations
- The white cell count, ESR or CRP may be raised
- Antistaphylococcal titres may be elevated
- Histology may show only reactive new bone formation but organisms are frequently identified

Management Chronic infection is rarely eradicated with antibiotics alone. Bed rest and dressing the sinus give symptomatic relief during an acute flare. Surgery is indicated if there are significant symptoms combined with evidence of a sequestrum or other necrotic bone. Dead bone can be identified at surgery, as it does not stain with methylene blue, and should be thoroughly debrided or excised. Irrigation can be continued postoperatively or gentamicin beads inserted. A bony defect is filled with cancellous bone graft and a skin defect with a myocutaneous flap. Vascularized bone grafts have been used for bony defects >6 cm with minimal soft tissue loss. Amputation is sometimes necessary.

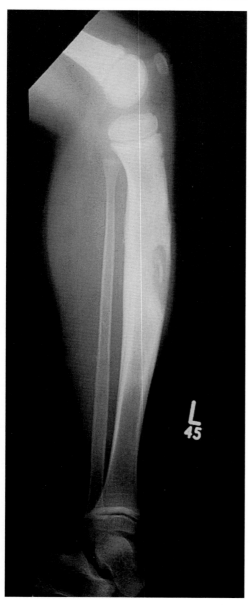

Fig 20.1 **Lateral lower leg.** An ovoid lucency is seen with a dense structure within it, the sequestrum. This is surrounded by a large area of sclerosis and mature periosteal reaction.

21 Cleidocranial dysostosis

Characteristics
- **Age range:** May be noted at any age
- **Gender:** M = F
- **Incidence:** 0.5 per 100 000 live births
- **Pathology:** Autosomal dominant inheritance

Clinical presentation Rarely, it may present at birth due to thoracic cage abnormalities. There is marked mobility of the shoulders, which are also 'droopy'. Dental eruption is delayed and the face appears small.

Radiology
Description
- ⚷ The clavicles are hypoplastic or absent
- Wormian bones and multiple extra teeth are present
- Midline defects and acroosteolysis are also associated
- Prognathism and a 'straight' mandible

Further imaging
- None

Non-radiological investigations
- None

Management Treatment is symptomatic.

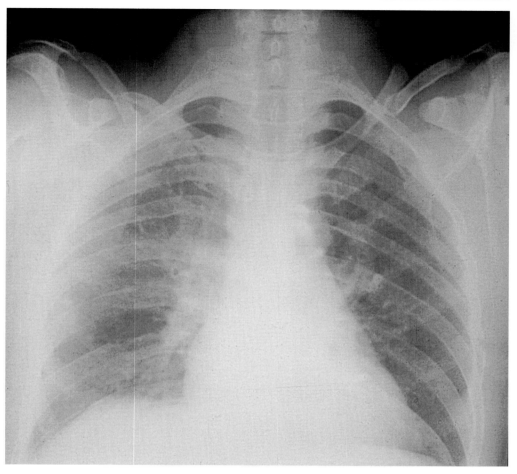

Fig 21.1 **AP chest.** Both clavicles are markedly hypoplastic.

22 Congenital vertical talus (rocker bottom foot)

Characteristics
- **Age range:** Infants
- **Gender:** M = F
- **Incidence:** Rare
- **Pathology:** Although most cases are idiopathic, some may be secondary to neuromuscular disorders, such as neural tube defects or arthrogryposis multiplex.

Clinical presentation A rounded prominence of the medial and plantar surfaces of the foot can usually be detected at birth. The calcaneum is in equinus and the sole is convex. There are deep creases on the dorsolateral aspect of the foot. It may be difficult to distinguish from severe pes planus.

Radiology
Description
- ☞ Talus is vertically orientated with an increased talocalcaneal angle
- Posterior dislocation of the navicular

Further imaging
- CT may help define anatomy

Non-radiological investigations
- None

Management It is difficult to correct and tends to recur. Open reduction of the talonavicular joint is usually required with navicular excision if the deformity is severe. In addition, 4–8-year-olds generally require soft tissue procedures and extraarticular subtalar arthrodesis. If the patient is older than 12 years then triple arthrodesis is the treatment of choice.

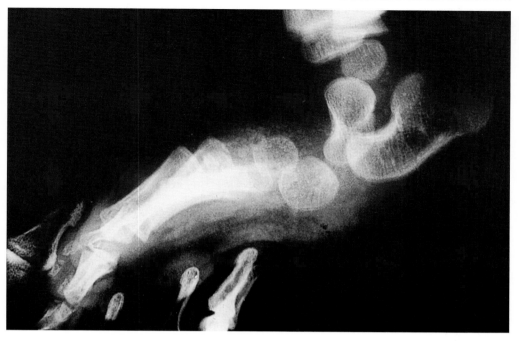

Fig 22.1 **Lateral foot.** Note the vertical position of the talus lying between the calcaneum and the navicular.

23 **Coxa vara**

Characteristics
- **Age range:** Infancy and early childhood
- **Gender:** M = F
- **Incidence:** 1 in 25 000
- **Pathology:** There may be avascular abnormality in the developing femoral neck. Some cases have been attributed to perinatal trauma.

Clinical presentation May present during ultrasonographic screening for DDH. The child may have a limp or waddling gait that may not be apparent until 3–4 years of age. 70% present with a painless limp, 5% with back and leg pain. The Trendelenburg sign is positive and decreased abduction and internal rotation are common. The affected leg is generally short, although rarely by more than 2 cm.

Radiology
Description
- 🗝 'Shepherd's crook' deformity of the femoral neck

- 🔔 Severe end of the spectrum is proximal focal femoral deficiency (PFFD) where variable amounts of the proximal femur are absent

Further imaging
- US or MR may be necessary to define the anatomy in PFFD

Non-radiological investigations
- None

Management Gait training and abductor muscle strengthening may help. Progressive shortening requires surgery to correct the deformity. A subtrochanteric valgus or oblique intertrochanteric osteotomy is performed. The latter allows correction of retroversion. The varus deformity does not recur, although there is usually some permanent shortening. PFFD may need a custom-built prosthesis.

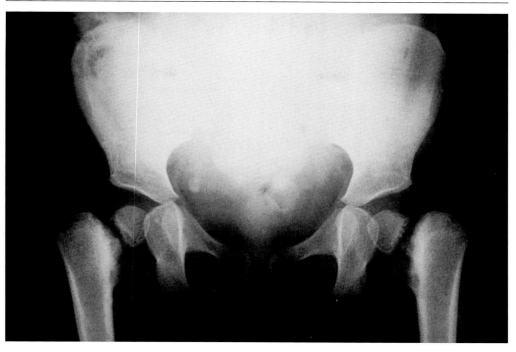

Fig 23.1 **AP pelvis.** There is bilateral, symmetrical abnormality of the proximal femoral metaphyses.

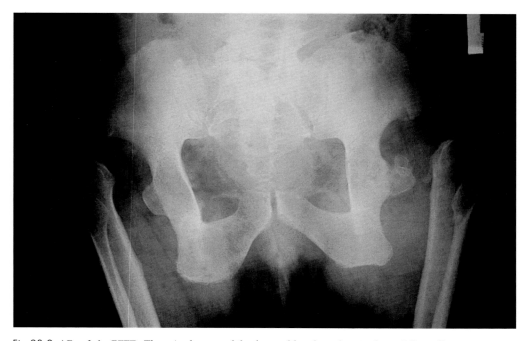

Fig 23.2 **AP pelvis, PFFD.** There is absence of the femoral heads and metaphyses bilaterally.

24 **Dermatomyositis**

Characteristics
- **Age range:** Bimodal; presents either in childhood or in the fourth to sixth decades
- **Gender:** M < F
- **Incidence:** Rare
- **Pathology:** Atrophy, oedema and necrosis occur in striated muscle but the aetiology is unknown.

Clinical presentation Muscle weakness, fatigue and pain. Dysphagia and rashes are also seen, together with arthritis and Raynaud's phenomenon. 🔔 It may be associated with an underlying neoplasm, particularly in the abdomen.

Radiology
Description
- 🗝 Calcification occurs in fascial planes, subcutaneous fat, tendons and fingertips

- Acroosteolysis
- Non-erosive arthropathy

Further imaging
- CT/US to look for underlying malignancy

Non-radiological investigations
- Serum creatinine phosphokinase is raised
- Muscle biopsy
- EMG

Management The acute form carries a poor prognosis. Symptomatic and supportive therapy are indicated, together with steroids.

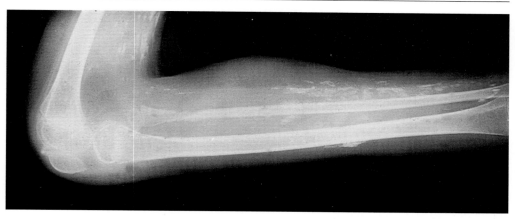

Fig 24.1 **Lateral forearm.** Sheets of calcification are seen in the subcutaneous tissues with marked muscle wasting.

25 Developmental dysplasia of the hip (DDH)

Characteristics
- **Age range:** Presents from birth
- **Gender:** M:F = 1:8
- **Incidence:** 1 in 500 births, higher for the first born
- **Pathology:** This is multifactorial. Known risk factors include breech presentation, where there is a short iliopsoas muscle. There may be excessive ligamentous laxity, possibly due to a maternal oestrogen effect. Heredity also plays a role with 6% of subsequent siblings and 12% of patient's children affected.

Clinical presentation Clinical screening is carried out at birth and again at 8 weeks for all children, looking for asymmetrical skin creases and a 'click' on hip abduction in flexion. 'At-risk' babies may be screened by US at 6 weeks. Late presentation occurs with walking problems, deformity or pain.

Radiology
Description
- US is the investigation of choice in the infant
- ⊶ The acetabular morphology and Graf α angle are evaluated (Fig 25.3). The latter should be over 59° in normal babies
- 50% or more of the femoral head should be contained within the acetabulum
- Subluxation or dislocation can be seen on dynamic scanning

Further imaging
- Plain films are necessary to evaluate the older infant
- The centre edge angle should be >15° in the normal hip
- Rarely, arthrography may be necessary

Non-radiological investigations
- None

Management Early diagnosis is treated by an abduction harness. The position of the hip should be checked by US every 2 weeks. Late diagnosis leads to permanent acetabular dysplasia and may require osteotomy or shelf formation to contain the femoral head. Very late presentation may be with premature OA and may need hip replacement.

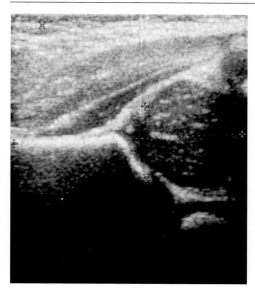

Fig 25.1 **Normal hip US.** Note the acetabular angle and containment of 50% of the unossified femoral head.

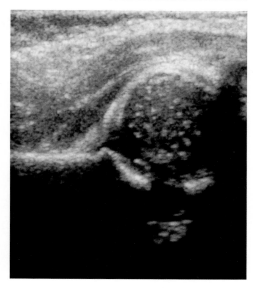

Fig 25.2 **Dysplastic hip US.** The acetabular angle is reduced and only one-third of the femoral head is contained.

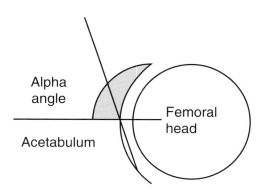

Fig 25.3 Lines used for calculating the Graf α angle.

26 **Diabetic arthropathy**

Characteristics
- **Age range:** Affects older patients with diabetes
- **Gender:** M = F
- **Incidence:** Common
- **Pathology:** Due to a combination of peripheral neuropathy and vascular insufficiency. Decreased pain sensation, reduced blood supply and continued use lead to uncontrolled damage and repair.

Clinical presentation Extensive foot ulceration is seen in conjunction with reduced foot pulses and reduced sensation.

Radiology
Description
- Soft tissue swelling may be associated with demineralization and subluxation
- Tissue defects due to ulceration may be obvious

- Small vessel calcification
- ☞ Repeated periosteal reaction and resorption lead to a dense, pointed bone

Further imaging
- Superadded infection may require white cell isotope scans or human immunoglobulin (HIG) scans to diagnose
- MRI accurately defines the extent of bony involvement

Non-radiological investigations
- None

Management Good control of the diabetes reduces the incidence of neurovascular complications. Trophic changes and infection may require debriding and eventual amputation.

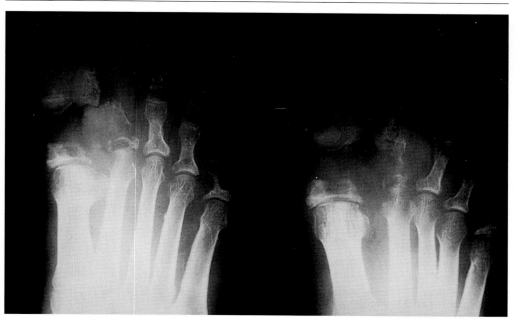

Fig 26.1 **DP foot.** Destructive changes are seen superimposed on a background of an increase in bone density. This is due to a combination of osteomyelitis, vascular insufficiency and peripheral neuropathy.

27 Diaphyseal aclasis (Multiple exostoses)

Characteristics
- **Age range:** Usually diagnosed between 2 and 10 years of age
- **Gender:** M:F = 2:1
- **Incidence:** Rare
- **Pathology:** Autosomal dominant inheritance. Ectopic cartilaginous rests in metaphyses lead to the formation of multiple osteochondromatous exostoses.

Clinical presentation There is a painless mass near a joint, although pain may occur from impingement on adjacent muscles, tendons, nerves or vessels. They may interfere with the mechanics of a joint or damage the growth plate, causing bowing and deformity. The lesions usually stop growing when the patient reaches skeletal maturity; onset of pain or further growth beyond this age is a sinister feature. When there are multiple exostoses the risk of malignant transformation is 6%.

Radiology
Description
- ☞ Multiple cartilage-capped exostoses at large joints, spine and pelvis
- As the bone grows they may 'migrate' up the shaft
- Broadening of the metaphyses
- Madelung deformity may develop
- Shortening of long bones
- ☀ Loss of definition and destruction of cartilage suggests malignant change

Further imaging
- MR and imaging-guided biopsy if malignant change is suspected

Non-radiological investigations
- Histology

Management Exostoses can be removed if symptomatic or for cosmetic reasons. Sarcomatous change is managed as necessary.

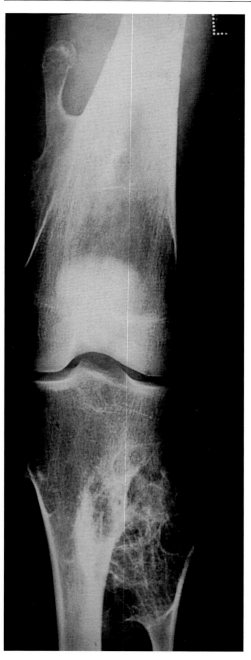

Fig 27.1 **AP knee.** Multiple cartilage-capped
exostoses are seen arising from the metaphyseal
areas, pointing away from the joints.

28 Diastematomyelia

Characteristics
- **Age range:** May present from birth to maturity, but commonly under the age of 5 years
- **Gender:** M = F
- **Incidence:** Rare
- **Pathology:** The spinal cord and/or filum terminale are split by a bony or fibrocartilaginous septum.

Clinical presentation Patients frequently present with associated abnormalities such as meningocoele, arachnoid cyst or cutaneous marker lesions – hair, naevus, lipoma or pit. They tend to present with neurological abnormalities, e.g. cavovarus foot deformity, paralytic valgus, trophic ulceration, short leg or small foot.

Radiology
Description
- Commonly associated with congenital scoliosis
- Increased interpediculate distance
- Vertebral bodies may appear normal or there may be spina bifida, hemivertebra, block vertebrae or fused posterior elements
- Bony spur can be identified in the spinal canal in 50%

Further imaging
- ☞ MR demonstrates a low conus, tethered cord and thickened filum terminale in addition to the split cord

Non-radiological investigations
- None

Management If there are neurological problems then surgery is indicated.

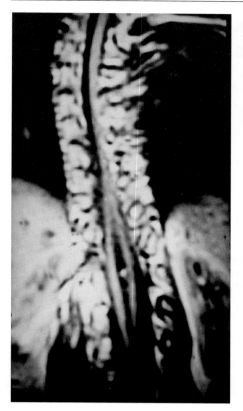

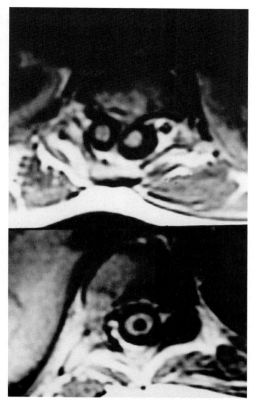

Fig 28.1 **Coronal T1-weighted MRI.** The cord is clearly shown to be split around a bony bar at the level of the thoracolumbar junction.

Fig 28.2 **Axial T1-weighted MRI.** This demonstrates the two separate components of the cord.

29 Diffuse idiopathic skeletal hyperostosis (DISH or Forrestier's disease)

Characteristics
- **Age range:** Middle age to elderly
- **Gender:** M > F
- **Incidence:** Uncommon
- **Pathology:** Ossification occurs at tendon and ligament insertions and particularly the anterior longitudinal ligament of the spinal column. There is an association with diabetes (10%) and hypertension (20%).

Clinical presentation Patients present with mild to moderate back pain, although significant stiffness is rare. There may be dysphagia if the cervical spine is affected. Spinal stenosis is rare.

Radiology
Description
- Florid spinal degenerative changes most often in the thoracic spine

- 🔑 Massive bridging osteophyte formation over four or more disc spaces
- Disc spaces are preserved
- New bone formation at entheses

Further imaging
- MR may be necessary to assess spinal stenosis

Non-radiological investigations
- HLA B27 negative

Management Symptomatic relief from antiinflammatory medication and physiotherapy.

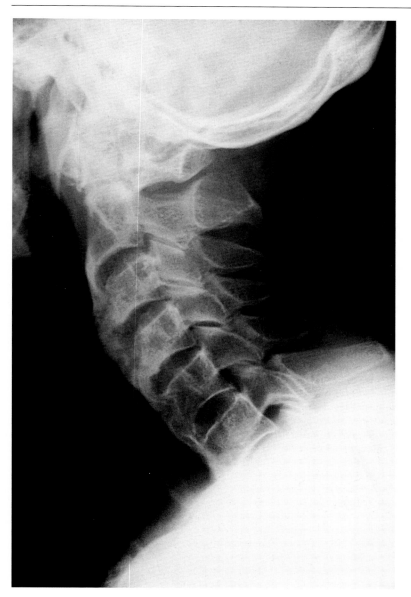

Fig 29.1 **Lateral cervical spine.** There is flowing osteophyte formation along the anterior longitudinal ligament.

30 **Disc herniation**

Characteristics
- **Age range:** Common at any age
- **Gender:** M = F
- **Incidence:** Asymptomatic herniation is seen in 21% of the population
- **Pathology:** Acute trauma to a healthy disc may cause rupture of the annulus fibrosus and prolapse of the nucleus. More commonly, there is progressive dehydration and reduction in discal volume as a normal part of ageing. This may lead to fissuring of the annulus. A disc bulge is a broad-based disc extrusion with a weak but intact annulus. Disc herniation is a focal protrusion of disc material through a ruptured annulus. When the posterior longitudinal ligament is torn there may be disc sequestration.

Clinical presentation The patient presents with pain, stiffness and muscle splinting at the affected spinal level. Pain radiates along the dermatome. There may be dermatomal sensory loss, weakness, muscle atrophy and loss of the relevant reflexes.

Radiology
Description
- 🔔 Plain film findings of loss of disc height and osteophyte formation do not correlate with the presence of significant disc herniation

Further imaging
- MR shows loss of disc signal on T2 scans as the first sign of degeneration due to dehydration
- 🔑 MR demonstrates the disc protrusion and will show if there is any thecal or nerve root compromise
- CT can show disc protrusion but uses ionizing radiation
- In the postoperative patient, gadolinium-enhanced MR demonstrates the difference between fibrosis and recurrent disc. The former enhances, the latter does not

Non-radiological investigations
- Electromyographic studies may lend supportive evidence

Management Discectomy may prove necessary for severe radicular symptoms or neurological loss, although many patients' symptoms are relieved by conservative treatment.

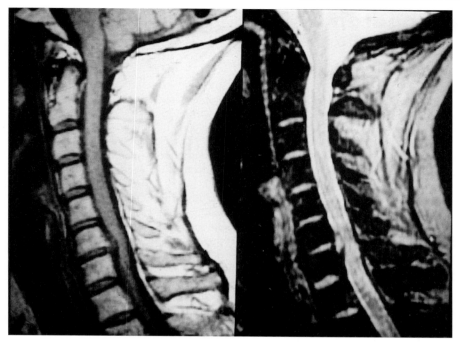

Fig 30.1 **T1- and T2-weighted sagittal cervical spine MR.** There is degenerative change at C6/7 with posterior osteophyte formation and a disc protrusion causing elevation of the posterior longitudinal ligaments. There is a suggestion of cord compression, which would need to be validated on the axial scan.

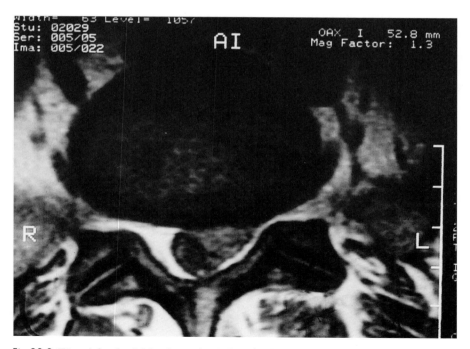

Fig 30.2 **T1-weighted axial lumbar spine MR.** A focal right paracentral disc herniation is seen.

31 **Enchondroma**

Characteristics

- **Age range:** Most often seen between the ages of 10 and 30 years but is seen at any age
- **Gender:** M = F
- **Incidence:** Common
- **Pathology:** There is persistence of cartilage islands in the metaphyses of bones formed by endochondral ossification. Microscopically hyaline cartilage is identified, often with a central area of degeneration or calcification. Multiple enchondromas are known as Ollier's disease (see p. 132).

Clinical presentation
Often asymptomatic and may present as an incidental finding on a radiograph or as a pathological fracture. The patient may notice a painless mass but pain in the absence of fracture is a sign of possible malignancy. ☀ Malignant transformation does occur in less than 2% of cases and very rarely in children. Lesions of the pelvis, femur and ribs are at higher risk. Most commonly affects tubular bones of the hands and feet.

Radiology
Description

- ☞ There is a well-defined lesion with reactive sclerosis

- Pathological fractures are common
- Small flecks of calcification can be seen inside the tumour
- Expansion and soft tissue deformities may result
- In a long bone a small area of dense chondroid calcification is seen

Further imaging

- Imaging-guided biopsy may be necessary
- Bone scan and MR may be used to confirm the benign nature of the lesion by absence of increased uptake or absence of high signal on T2-weighted scans

Non-radiological investigations

- Histology

Management
Curettage with or without bone graft is usually curative in children although there is a high rate of local recurrence in adults. Resection or curettage combined with cryosurgery have the highest success rate. Pathological fractures may require internal fixation but sometimes result in healing. ☀ It may be necessary to differentiate the appearance from low-grade chondrosarcoma, which may look very similar.

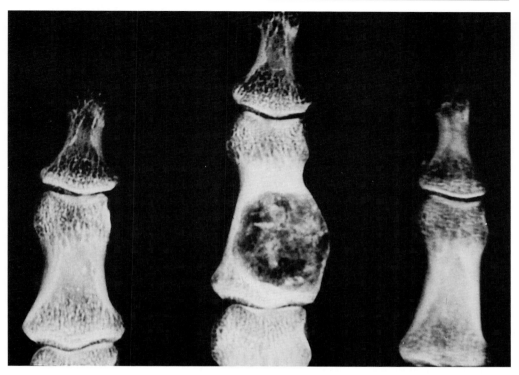

Fig 31.1 **DP phalanges.** An expansile lesion is seen at the base of the middle finger, middle phalanx. This is well defined and contains multiple chondroid calcifications.

32 Ewing's sarcoma

Characteristics
- **Age range:** Peak incidence is in the second decade
- **Gender:** M:F = 2:1
- **Incidence:** 4–10% of all bone tumours; the second most common primary bone tumour of childhood
- **Pathology:** Infiltration by malignant round cells; these are closely packed with an indistinct cell membrane

Clinical presentation The patient complains of pain, swelling, erythema and induration; 25% of patients present with systemic signs such as fever, anorexia and weight loss. Sixty percent occur in the long bones (25% in the femur) and soft tissue extension is common. In the older age group (>20 years) lesions arise in the flat bones and are termed round cell or peripheral neuroectodermal tumours. In the ribs it is called an Askin tumour and has a significantly better prognosis.

Radiology
Description
- Diaphyseal or metadiaphyseal
- ☞ Extensive lytic lesion which is permeative or fusiform
- Periosteal reaction which classically has a lamellated 'onion-skin' appearance
- Associated soft tissue mass
- No tumour bone formation

Further imaging
- ☀ Bone scan shows metastases in up to 30% at presentation
- Chest CT for distant staging
- MRI for local staging
- Imaging-guided biopsy

Non-radiological investigations
- Histology
- Anaemia, leucocytosis and a raised ESR
- Chromosomal analysis reveals translocation of the long arms of chromosomes 11 and 22

Management Five-year survival is 60–75%. All patients require chemotherapy and the lesion is radiosensitive although when used alone, the local recurrence rate is up to 30%. Surgery plays an increasing role in the management of Ewing's sarcoma, generally after initial chemotherapy. The best results are achieved with the combination of all three methods of treatment.

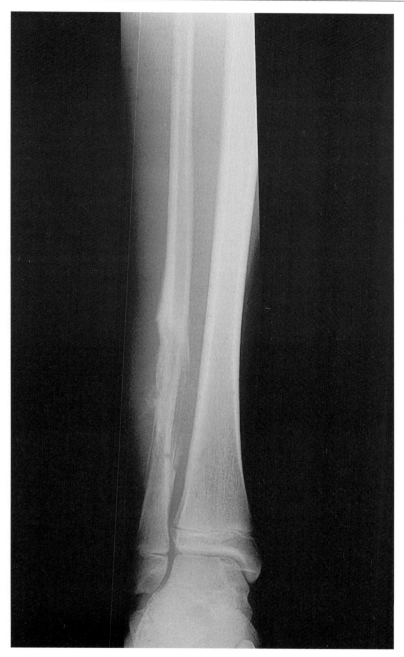

Fig 32.1 **AP lower leg.** There is a lytic lesion in the distal fibula which demonstrates the classic 'onion-skin' periosteal reaction on the medial side.

33 **Fibrous dysplasia**

Characteristics
- **Age range:** Most often presents between the ages of 3 and 15 years
- **Gender:** M = F
- **Incidence:** Monostotic disease is fairly common but polyostotic disease is rare
- **Pathology:** There is a congenital abnormality of the bone-forming mesenchyme. It can affect one bone (monostotic), one limb (monomelic) or multiple bones (polyostotic). Histology shows fibrous tissue with areas of osteoid and woven bone.

Clinical presentation Small, solitary lesions are asymptomatic and found incidentally. Larger lesions may present with pain or a pathological fracture when cystic degeneration has occurred. Cherubism is a familial form, which is confined to the facial bones and causes disfigurement. Polyostotic fibrous dysplasia is seen in association with precocious puberty and excess pigmentation in Albright–McCune syndrome. ⚠ Rarely aneurysmal bone cysts or even malignant change may occur as a secondary phenomenon, usually in polyostotic disease.

Radiology
Description
- Lesions have a dense sclerotic rim – the 'rind sign'
- Abnormal modelling and some expansion may be seen
- 🔑 Matrix has 'ground glass' calcification
- Cystic change may rarely occur

Further imaging
- Bone scanning gives variable results, from hot to cold spots
- MR demonstrates secondary changes well but the fibrous tissue is normally of low signal on all sequences
- Imaging-guided biopsy

Non-radiological investigations
- Histology

Management Small lesions need no treatment. Large lesions and those that have fractured can be curetted and grafted but recurrence is high. The only definitive treatment is wide local excision, radical resection or amputation, although this is seldom necessary.

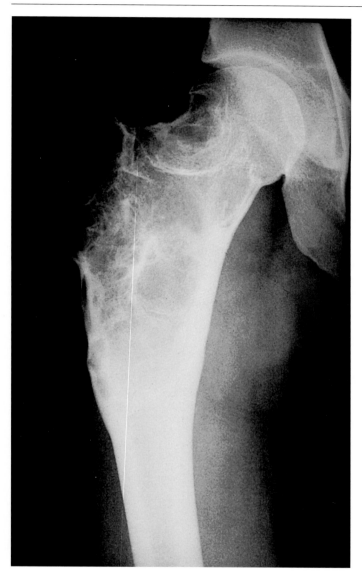

Fig 33.1 **AP hip.** There is modelling deformity in association with mixed lucency in a background of 'ground glass'. The lesion has a well-defined rim (rind sign).

34 **Fluorosis**

Characteristics
- **Age range:** May present at any age
- **Gender:** M = F
- **Incidence:** Rare in the UK, endemic in some countries where drinking water is overfluorinated
- **Pathology:** Deposition of fluoroapatite crystals in bone. There is presumed to be an overactivity of parathyroid hormone leading to increased deposition and reduced resorption of bone.

Clinical presentation Mottling of tooth enamel and anaemia. The bone changes are rarely symptomatic but may produce pain.

Radiology
Description
- ⚬— Generalized increase in bone density, predominantly in the axial skeleton
- 'Whiskering' and 'feathering' at soft tissue insertions into bone
- Florid osteophyte formation, particularly in the spine
- Affected children may develop bone deformity

Further imaging
- None

Non-radiological investigations
- Serum calcium and phosphate are usually normal

Management None is usually needed.

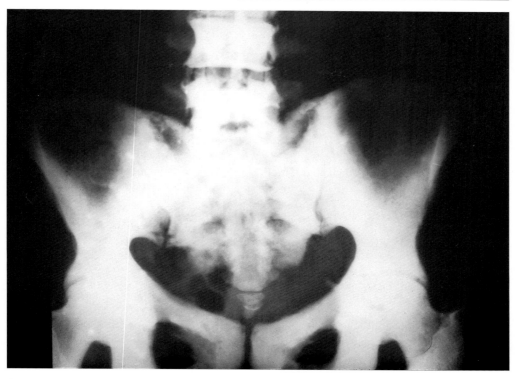

Fig 34.1 **AP pelvis.** There is generalized increase in bone density with some feathering at the bone margins.

35 Gaucher's disease

Characteristics
- **Age range:** Present in childhood or adult life
- **Gender:** M = F
- **Incidence:** Rare
- **Pathology:** Autosomal recessive. It is most prevalent in patients of Ashkenazi origin (Central and East European). There is an inborn error of glycosphingolipid metabolism – lack of β glycosidase enzyme. Cerebrosides accumulate in reticuloendothelial cells and other tissues.

Clinical presentation Patients often present with haematological problems (anaemia, thrombocytopenia) and/or splenomegaly. Skeletal involvement – bone pain, loss of movement in a large joint – is not related to the extent of visceral disease. Acute crises mimic osteomyelitis or septic arthritis. Pathological fracture is rare. Any bone may be involved, though major disability is usually secondary to AVN of femoral or humeral heads. Infantile Gaucher's may present with neurological problems – neck rigidity, dysphagia, catatonia, hyperreflexia and mental retardation.

Radiology
Description
- Generalized loss of bone density
- Coarse trabecular pattern
- Lytic lesions or well-defined moth-eaten appearance may mimic metastases
- Erlenmeyer flask deformity of distal femur and proximal tibia
- Pathological fractures and secondary joint degeneration
- Cortex thinned, scalloped or thickened
- AVN, particularly of femoral head
- Spine is osteopenic with wedge deformity or H-shaped vertebrae

Further imaging
- US to look for an enlarged spleen with hypoechoic foci
- CT to demonstrate nodules and low-attenuation lesions in the spleen
- CXR and HRCT of the lung show diffuse reticulonodular lung infiltrates

Non-radiological investigations
- Serum angiotensin-converting enzyme and tartrate-resistant acid phosphatase levels are often elevated
- Mildly elevated ESR and leucocytes in bone crisis

Management Historically involved blood product infusions, partial or total splenectomy, analgesia and even bone marrow transplantation in rapidly progressive disease. Hyperbaric oxygen can be used for acute crises. Now, treatment generally consists of enzyme replacement therapy. Avascular necrosis may require surgery.

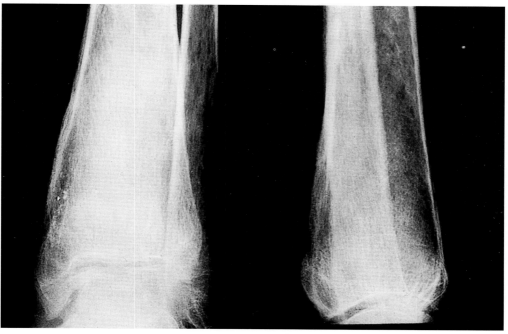

Fig 35.1 **AP and lateral ankle.** There is modelling deformity of the distal tibia with a mottled appearance of the medulla and a thinned cortex.

36 Giant cell tumour

Characteristics
- **Age range:** 80% occur between the ages of 20 and 40 years
- **Gender:** M < F
- **Incidence:** 4.2% of all primary bone tumours, 21% of benign lesions
- **Pathology:** A lesion of uncertain origin occurring in mature bone. It is aggressive and locally recurrent but has low metastatic potential. Macroscopically it has a reddish, fleshy appearance and the histology shows an abundance of multinucleate giant cells. 🔔 15% become frankly malignant after local recurrence.

Clinical presentation Patients present with pain at or near a joint, slight swelling, an effusion or pathological fracture; 75% occur around the knee but other common sites are the proximal humerus and distal radius. Multiple lesions are rare.

Radiology
Description
- 🔑 A lytic lesion is contiguous with an articular or apophyseal surface
- There is an intermediate zone of transition
- A breach in the cortex is common
- Matrix mineralization occurs very rarely

Further imaging
- MR for local anatomy
- Imaging-guided biopsy

Non-radiological investigations
- Histology

Management 'Benign' lesions are treated by curettage, with or without bone grafting. Aggressive and recurrent lesions are treated by en bloc resection with bone grafting, cement insertion or prosthetic replacement. Cryosurgery has been used and radiotherapy is considered when surgical excision is not technically possible. Amputation is reserved for massive recurrence or malignant transformation.

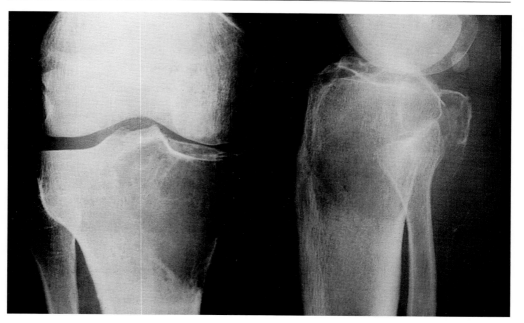

Fig 36.1 **AP knee.** There is a relatively well-defined lytic lesion in the medial aspect of the tibial plateau. This extends as far as the articular surface. Note that there is some diffuse osteopenia in the adjacent femoral condyle. There is no evidence of pathological fracture or soft tissue extension.

37 **Gout**

Characteristics
- **Age range:** Occurs from the fifth decade onwards
- **Gender:** M:F = 20:1
- **Incidence:** Three cases per 1000 population
- **Pathology:** A metabolic disorder resulting in hyperuricaemia and deposition of monosodium urate monohydrate in synovial fluid. Primary gout is due to an inherited enzyme defect. Secondary gout may be due to excessive nucleoprotein breakdown, as in haematological disorders, or renal failure. Crystals are deposited in the synovium and carried to the articular surface where they cause an intense inflammatory reaction with pannus formation. This erodes cartilage and bone. Tophi consist of sodium urate crystals and are deposited in bone, cartilage, synovium, ligaments, bursae and subcutaneous tissue.

Clinical presentation The patient presents with acute attacks of inflammatory arthritis. The commonest site is the first MTP joint (75% of cases) and other small joints of the hands and feet; it may also affect large joints, including the sacroiliac joints and the spine. Extraarticular manifestations include renal failure, urate stones and cardiac disease.

Radiology
Description
- Asymmetrical and random distribution
- Joint effusion and soft tissue swelling
- Uniform joint space narrowing
- Juxtaarticular, 'punched out' erosions
- Normal bone density except where there has been severe persistent pain
- Tophi result in a dense soft tissue mass; bony destruction may occur remote from the articular surface

Further imaging
- None

Non-radiological investigations
- Serum urate is elevated and urate crystals are present in the synovial fluid

Management Acute attacks are treated with antiinflammatory agents. Long-term prophylaxis is provided by allopurinol.

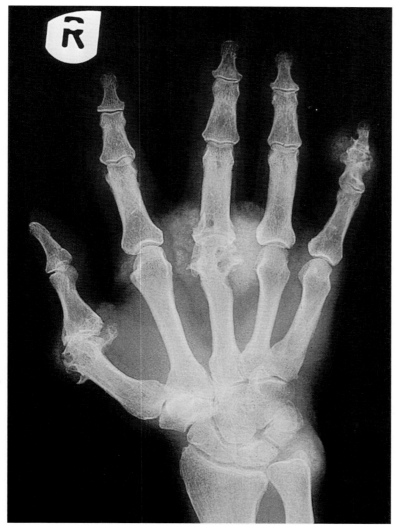

Fig 37.1 **DP hand.** There are multiple well-defined, juxtaarticular erosions. In addition, there is soft tissue swelling due to tophus formation.

38 **Haemangioma**

Characteristics
- **Age range:** May present at any age, depending on the type of lesion
- **Gender:** M = F
- **Incidence:** Common
- **Pathology:** They may be true neoplasms, hamartomas or vascular malformations. Capillary haemangiomas are the most common; others are cavernous, venous or arteriovenous. Rarely, they may become malignant.

Clinical presentation A capillary haemangioma is the common reddish 'birthmark' seen on the skin. A cavernous haemangioma is a sponge-like collection of vessels leading to a purple mark overlying a soft subcutaneous mass. Lesions may extend into the fascia, muscle or bone or may affect an entire limb, leading to hypertrophy. Entirely subcutaneous or bony lesions may present as a mass or with pain.

Radiology
Description
- A soft tissue mass may contain spherical calcifications – phleboliths

- Affected bone may show large vascular channels
- ☞ US with Doppler evaluation can often demonstrate blood flow and the extent of the lesion

Further imaging
- MR or angiography may be required to demonstrate the feeding and draining vessels
- Radiological embolization may be appropriate

Non-radiological investigations
- None

Management Treatment is only required if there is discomfort or disability and recurrence is common after local excision. Lesions may also be pretreated by embolization.

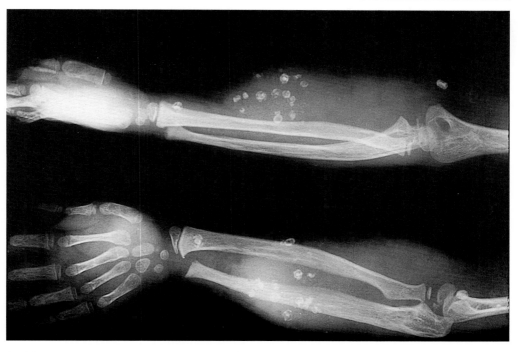

Fig 38.1 **AP and lateral forearm.** There is enlargement of the soft tissues and multiple phleboliths are seen.

39 Haemochromatosis

Characteristics
- **Age range:** Middle age
- **Gender:** M:F = 10:1
- **Incidence:** Rare
- **Pathology:** Haemosiderin is deposited in the soft tissues either because of a genetic abnormality or as a result of iron overload. ⚠ This also occurs in the viscera, leading to liver, pancreatic and gonadal failure. Calcium pyrophosphate is deposited in the synovium as well as haemosiderin. Deposition in articular cartilage leads to arthropathy. Primary disease is due to a gene with autosomal recessive transmission; secondary disease is due to excessive iron absorption or ingestion.

Clinical presentation The syndrome is known as 'bronzed diabetes'. In addition to cirrhosis, cardiac failure and skin pigmentation, patients present with an inflammatory arthropathy with joint pain, swelling and stiffness.

Radiology
Description
- Affected joints show mild osteopenia
- Chondrocalcinosis
- 🔑 Predominantly affects the MCP joints with 'hook' formation of the metacarpal heads

Further imaging
- ⚠ Abdominal US may reveal hepatoma in up to 30%
- Brain MR shows decreased signal in the anterior pituitary from iron deposition

Non-radiological investigations
- Raised serum iron
- Liver biopsy

Management Death usually occurs from heart (30%) or liver (25%) failure. Management is by therapeutic phlebotomy or use of a chelating agent to reduce iron absorption.

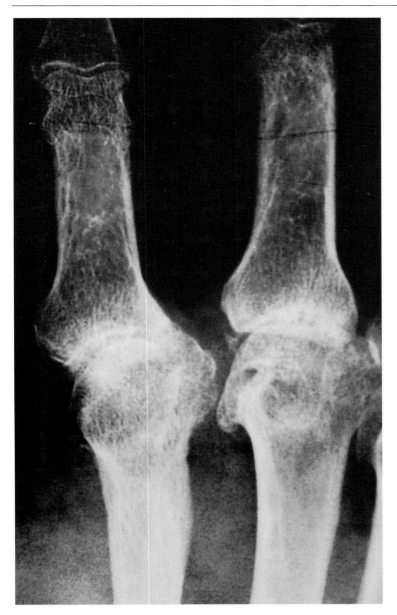

Fig 39.1 **DP MCP joints.** There is advanced degenerative change with hook formation at the MC heads.

40 **Haemophilia**

Characteristics

- **Age range:** May present at any age but most commonly in childhood
- **Gender:** Males and XO females only
- **Incidence:** 1 in 10 000
- **Pathology:** X-linked recessive inheritance. There is a deficiency of clotting factor VIII (levels less than 5% of normal lead to mild disease, less than 1% severe disease). Frequent spontaneous joint and muscle haemorrhages lead to synovial inflammation and subsynovial fibrosis. Vascular pannus gradually erodes articular cartilage and bone, causing premature osteoarthritis.

Clinical presentation There is pain and swelling due to spontaneous haemarthroses which occur most commonly in the knee, usually after the child has begun to walk. Joint contractures are common. Acute bleeding into muscles occurs less frequently but may compress peripheral nerves, resulting in neuropraxia.

Radiology

Description

- Intraarticular haemorrhage commonly in knee, ankle and elbow
- Soft tissue swelling with large epiphyses

- Diffuse osteoporosis
- Erosion of articular surface and subchondral cyst formation
- Widening of the intercondylar notch of knee
- Soft tissue haemosiderin deposition
- 🔔 Haemorrhage into bone or muscle may produce a 'haemophilic pseudotumour' – single or multiple intramedullary cystic expansile lesions, which may have an associated soft tissue mass
- Secondary degenerative change

Further imaging

- CT to demonstrate pseudotumour extent
- MR will show haemorrhage of varying age

Non-radiological investigations

- 🔑 Factor VIII levels are reduced in the blood

Management Clotting factor replacement and pain relief. The affected joint or muscle is splinted in the acute phase and then movement is encouraged. Physiotherapy and intermittent splinting for contractures. Surgery may be indicated: tendon lengthening, osteotomy, arthrodesis or arthroplasty.

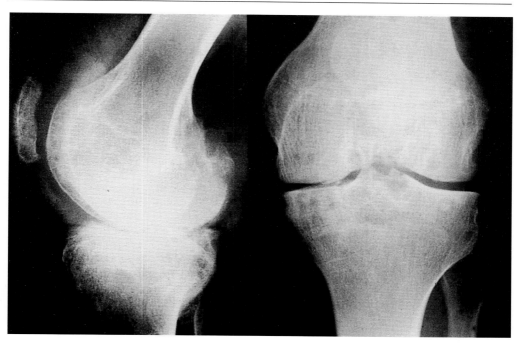

Fig 40.1 **AP and lateral knee.** There is reduction in the joint space and subchondral cyst formation. Soft tissue density is seen due to haemosiderin deposits following repeated haemarthroses.

41 Hurler's syndrome (mucopolysaccharidosis I)

Characteristics
- **Age range:** Presents in the first 2–3 years of life
- **Gender:** M = F
- **Incidence:** Very rare
- **Pathology:** There is a defect of lysosomal α-L-iduronidase in all tissues which leads to an accumulation of mucopolysaccharides in mesenchymal and parenchymal tissues and lipids in neural tissues.

Clinical presentation
The patient is of short stature with a coarse facies and hazy corneas. There may be kyphosis and a thoracolumbar gibbus, stiff joints, hepatosplenomegaly and mental retardation. ☀ Cardiac and respiratory complications cause death in childhood.

Radiology
Description
- Thickened calvarium with deformity due to premature fusion of sagittal and lambdoid sutures
- J-shaped sella
- Small facial bones, large mandible and dental anomalies
- Undertubulation of bones with a wavy contour and tapered ends
- 🔑 'Trident' hands with proximal tapering of MCs
- Oval vertebrae with an inferior beak
- Flared iliac wings which taper towards the acetabulum

Further imaging
- US, CT or MR may show hydrocephalus
- US for hepatosplenomegaly

Non-radiological investigations
- There is an excess of dermatan and heparan sulphate in the urine
- Lysosomal α-L-iduronidase is absent in cultured fibroblasts

Management
There is no specific treatment, except for the complications.

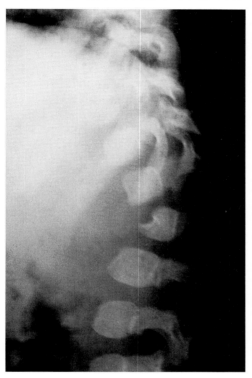

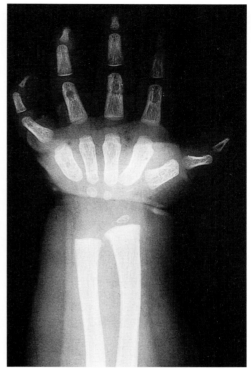

Fig 41.1 **Lateral spine.** There is inferior beaking of the vertebra with an associated angular kyphosis.

Fig 41.2 **DP hand.** There is a degree of undertubulation of the hand bones and retardation of the appearance of epiphyseal ossification centres.

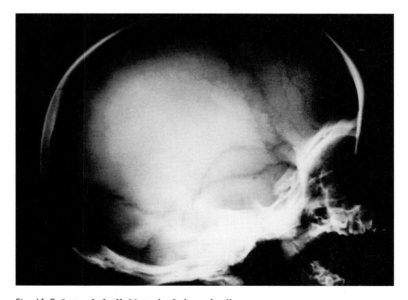

Fig 41.3 **Lateral skull.** Note the J-shaped sella.

42 **Hydatid disease**

Characteristics
- **Age range:** Predominantly adults
- **Gender:** M = F
- **Incidence:** Bone involvement is rare
- **Pathology:** It is caused by ingestion of echinococcus tapeworm cysts by contact with dog faeces or infected meat. Cysts contain many scolices, which pass into the blood and may lead to the formation of hydatid cysts, usually in the lung or liver. It is rare in the developed world.

Clinical presentation Patients present with pain and swelling or with a pathological fracture or spinal cord compression. Vertebrae, pelvis, ribs and femur are most commonly affected. It is most common in rural sheep-farming regions.

Radiology
Description
- 🔑 Multiple well-defined cysts of varying size are seen
- Endosteal scalloping and expansion

Further imaging
- MR and CT show fluid-filled cysts
- Imaging-guided biopsy may be appropriate

Non-radiological investigations
- Serology – the Casoni complement fixation test

Management For non-osseous lesions surgical excision is required if cysts are symptomatic. There is controversy over the value of radiological intervention. Albendazole is moderately effective at destroying the parasite. Bone cysts do not heal and may require curettage and bone grafting; the cavity is irrigated with hypertonic saline at the time of surgery.

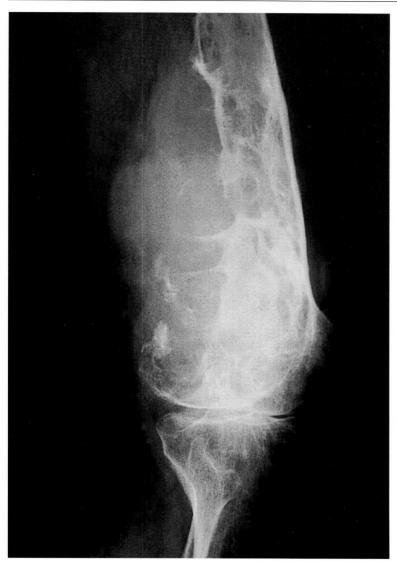

Fig 42.1 **Lateral knee.** The distal femur contains multiple lytic lesions. There is a suggestion of a soft tissue mass and a posterior break in the cortex but no new bone formation.

43 Hyperparathyroidism (HPT)

Characteristics
- **Age range:** Most commonly presents in the third and fourth decades
- **Gender:** M:F = 1:3
- **Incidence:** 25 cases of primary HPT per 100 000 per year
- **Pathology:** 87% of cases are due to a parathyroid adenoma producing excess parathyroid hormone (PTH). Secondary HPT is due to parathyroid hyperplasia consequent on prolonged hypocalcaemia. The tertiary form arises when secondary HPT results in autonomous PTH production.

Clinical presentation Bone lesions are seen in 25–40% of patients but many patients are found to be hypercalcaemic on routine blood testing. Raised serum calcium may lead to muscle weakness, abdominal pain, polyuria, renal colic, bone pain and pathological fractures. Secondary HPT leads to soft tissue calcification. Primary HPT rarely is associated with multiple endocrine adenoma syndromes I and II.

Radiology
Description
- Loss of bone density
- Subperiosteal bone resorption
- Erosions around the iliac crests, sacroiliac joints and acromioclavicular joints
- Widespread skull abnormality – 'pepper pot' appearance
- Loss of the lamina dura around the teeth
- Acroosteolysis
- 'Brown tumours' – multiple well-defined lytic lesions which are subarticular or metaphyseal

Further imaging
- Thyroid US, neck CT or MR to look for an adenoma
- Venous sampling to search for the source of ectopic PTH production

Non-radiological investigations
- PTH is raised
- Alkaline phosphatase is usually raised

Management Primary HPT requires surgical resection of the adenoma. Secondary HPT requires treatment of the underlying condition. Tertiary HPT also requires surgery.

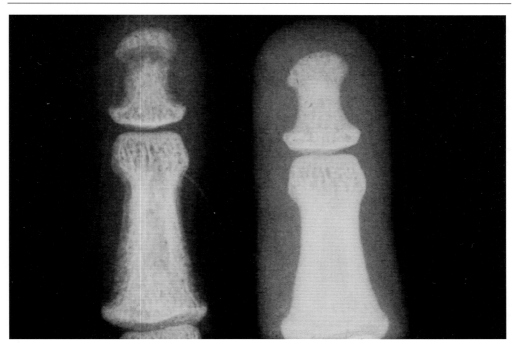

Fig 43.1 **DP phalanges compared with normal phalanges.** There is acroosteolysis, loss of bone density and subcortical tunnelling.

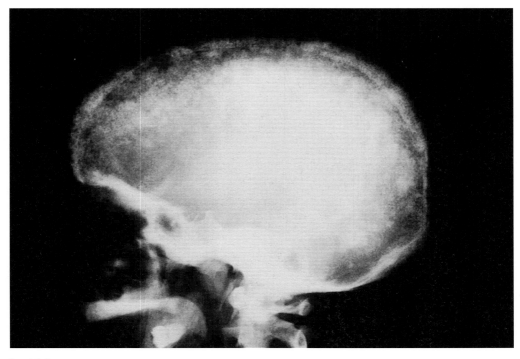

Fig 43.2 **Lateral skull.** There is mixed sclerosis and lucency in the skull vault.

44 Hypertrophic osteoarthropathy (HOA)

Characteristics
- **Age range:** Reflects the age range of the underlying pathology
- **Gender:** M = F
- **Incidence:** Rare
- **Pathology:** Underlying conditions such as thoracic neoplasia, chronic lung infection, congenital heart disease, chronic gastrointestinal or hepatic inflammation, nasopharyngeal or pancreatic carcinoma produce neurogenic peripheral vasodilatation, via the vagus. Vasodilators are released which are not metabolized by the lungs, possibly due to small AV shunts.

Clinical presentation Commonly seen at the wrists, hands, knees and ankles; the patient may develop pain and swelling at these sites and clubbing.

Radiology
Description
- ☞ Symmetrical diametaphyseal periosteal reaction
- Cortical thickening
- Soft tissue swelling may be seen at the terminal phalanges

Further imaging
- ☀ CXR may show the underlying cause, commonly a bronchial neoplasm
- Bone scan shows symmetrical uptake of tracer in a periosteal distribution
- US, mammography, CT or MRI to look for a primary

Non-radiological investigations
- None

Management Treatment of the underlying condition. Vagotomy may lead to regression.

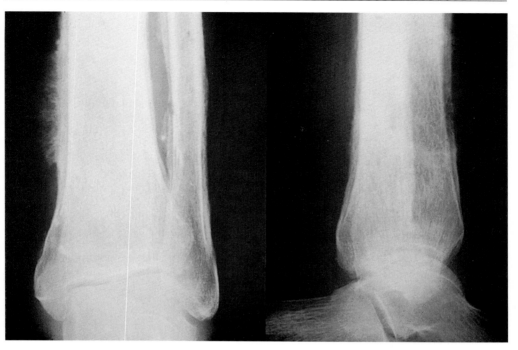

Fig 44.1 **AP and lateral ankle.** There is a florid periosteal reaction affecting all the bones circumferentially.

45 Infective discitis

Characteristics
- **Age range:** Children aged 2–6 years or adults
- **Gender:** M = F
- **Incidence:** Not rare
- **Pathology:** In children, haematogenous spread to the disc via arteries that continue to supply discs up to maturity. In adults, secondary to instrumentation or vertebral osteomyelitis once the endplate has been destroyed, i.e. by local spread. Most commonly due to Staphylococcus species.

Clinical presentation Classically a child with a 2–4-week history of back pain who may refuse to stand or walk and the spine may be held in a rigid hyperlordosis. Low-grade fever may be present although systemic features are usually mild. It most commonly occurs in the lower lumbar spine.

Radiology
Description
- ✵ Early plain films may be normal
- ☛ Loss of disc height with destruction of the endplates
- Gradual progression to destruction of the vertebral bodies
- May heal with ankylosis

Further imaging
- MR shows high signal in the disc on T2 weighting and high signal at the endplates, extending into the vertebral bodies
- Gadolinium may give enhancement of an abscess wall around the infective focus
- Bone scan will be hot prior to plain films being abnormal
- Imaging-guided biopsy

Non-radiological investigations
- ESR or CRP is raised in 90% of cases although the white cell count is often normal
- Blood cultures may grow an organism
- Biopsy material is usually culture negative

Management Bed rest and spinal immobilization with a cast. Systemic antibiotics are used if symptoms do not resolve rapidly or in cases with systemic signs of infection. The results are generally good: 25% of patients go on to spontaneous interbody fusion, 30% achieve restoration of disc height, 50% are left with a mild scoliosis. Premature degenerative change is common.

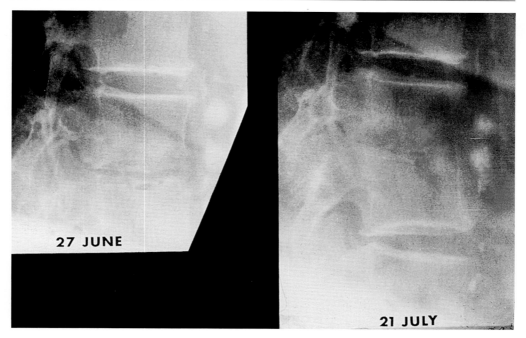

Fig 45.1 Lateral spine. The initial film shows reduction in the disc space with slight blurring of the adjacent endplates. By the second film there has been extensive destruction of the endplates and evidence of destruction of the superior parts of the vertebral bodies.

46 Irritable hip

Characteristics
- **Age range:** 5–10 years, with a peak incidence aged 6
- **Gender:** M:F = 2:1
- **Incidence:** Common
- **Pathology:** Sixty-five percent have a history of an associated viral illness and there is a non-specific inflammatory reaction of unknown aetiology.

Clinical presentation It is the most common non-traumatic cause of an acute limp which develops over 1–2 days. There may be an associated mild pyrexia.

Radiology
Description
- Plain films do not diagnose or exclude a hip effusion but may be indicated to exclude other pathology
- ☞ US shows elevation of the joint capsule by an effusion which is hypoechoic
- ☀ The appearance of a septic arthritis of the hip may be identical

Further imaging
- US-guided aspiration of the effusion

Non-radiological investigations
- MC+S of the effusion

Management Aspirating the effusion leads to rapid symptomatic relief, as may keeping the child non-weight bearing. There is complete recovery within a few weeks.

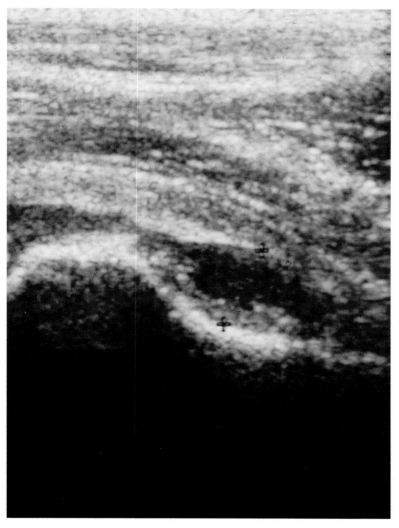

Fig 46.1 **Longitudinal US of the hip in a child.** Note the elevation of the capsule by hypoechoic fluid. The unfused physis can be clearly seen.

47 Juvenile chronic arthritis

Characteristics
- **Age range:** Children
- **Gender:** M > F, generally depending on the type
- **Incidence:** 1 per 1000
- **Pathology:** A non-infective inflammatory joint disorder of greater than 3 months duration in children less than 16 years of age. Similar to rheumatoid arthritis; a synovial inflammation secondary to an abnormal immune response leading to fibrosis and ankylosis but cartilage erosion is less marked than in rheumatoid. Children have a genetic predisposition.

Clinical presentation May present in a number of ways. Still's disease (15%) – a systemic disease in children less than 3 years of age with fevers, rash, malaise, lymphadenopathy and hepatosplenomegaly. Joint stiffness and swelling may not present until months later. Pauciarticular arthritis (60–70%) – usually less than 6 years old. Few joints are involved and there is no systemic illness but iridocyclitis occurs in 50%. Polyarticular arthritis (10%) – older children, classically affecting the temporomandibular joints and cervical spine. The hands and wrists are often affected. Seronegative spondyloarthritis (5–10%) – older children with sacroiliitis and spondylitis, a form of juvenile ankylosing spondylitis.

Radiology
Description
- There is soft tissue swelling and osteopenia

- Erosions are not often seen
- 🔑 There is epiphyseal overgrowth but premature closure of the physes
- Fusion across joints occurs, particularly in the cervical spine
- Bones may remain small throughout life

Further imaging
- MR of the cervical spine may be necessary for later symptoms

Non-radiological investigations
- Rheumatoid factor usually negative
- White cell count and ESR raised in systemic form
- HLA B27 positive in seronegative spondyloarthritis
- Joint aspiration and synovial biopsy may be necessary to establish the diagnosis

Management General treatment includes the use of gold or penicillamine; steroids are reserved for severe systemic disease or iridocyclitis resistant to topical treatment. Local treatment includes night splints and exercise to prevent deformity. Fixed deformities may require surgery and eroded joints may need replacing (often custom made). Five to ten percent of those affected are severely disabled and require treatment into adult life and approximately 3% die prematurely, usually secondary to renal failure (e.g. amyloidosis) or overwhelming infection.

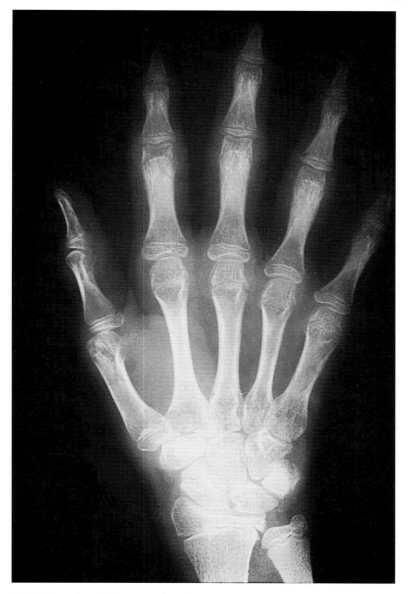

Fig 47.1 **DP hand.** There is profound periarticular osteopenia and some soft tissue swelling.

48 Langerhans cell histiocytosis

Characteristics
- **Age range:** Most often seen in 5–10-year-olds
- **Gender:** M:F = 3:2
- **Incidence:** 1 in 200 000, or 40 cases pa in UK
- **Pathology:** There is a proliferation of reticulum cells with accumulation of lipids. Histiocytes fuse to form giant cells containing Langerhans bodies.

Clinical presentation A spectrum of disease exists, from haemorrhage and purpura with anaemia and failure to thrive to more benign lesions presenting with bone pain. Diabetes insipidus, exophthalmia and intractable otitis media are associated. A skin rash may be seen. ☀ Acute forms have a high mortality with the more benign form being self-limiting.

Radiology
Description
- Solitary or multiple lesions predominantly in the axial skeleton and skull
- Intermediate/narrow zone of transition

- Skull lesions may show a 'geographical' or 'bevelled' margin
- May occur in the mandible, giving rise to 'floating' teeth
- ☛ Dense collapse of vertebral bodies; the 'silver dollar' sign is seen
- Spontaneous healing produces ill-defined sclerotic lesions

Further imaging
- Imaging-guided biopsy
- Bone scanning to look for other lesions
- CXR may show a reticulonodular pattern
- Abdominal US to look for hepatosplenomegaly and lymphadenopathy

Non-radiological investigations
- Raised ESR
- Pancytopenia or eosinophilia

Management Curettage or radiotherapy of bone lesions. Chemotherapy for more aggressive forms. The prognosis depends on the extent of disease and which organs are involved.

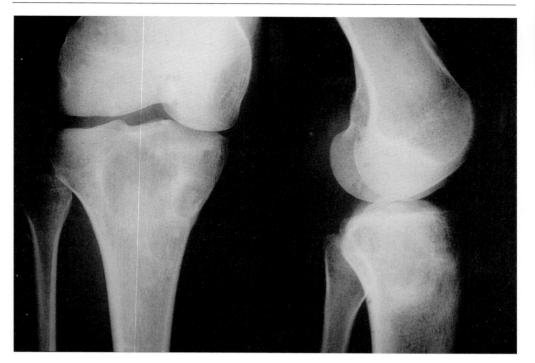

Fig 48.1 **AP and lateral knee.** Multiple well-defined lesions with sclerotic margins are noted in the proximal tibia. These are partly lytic but with an expanding zone of sclerosis consistent with healing of the lesion.

49 **Lead poisoning**

Characteristics
- **Age range:** Any age from infancy
- **Gender:** M = F
- **Incidence:** Very rare
- **Pathology:** There is excessive ingestion of lead, commonly from water pipes, paint, cosmetics or exhaust fumes. It is concentrated in the metaphyses of growing bones.

Clinical presentation Encephalopathy, abdominal pain or peripheral neuritis. Chronic exposure may lead to intellectual impairment.

Radiology
Description
- In children, cerebral oedema may lead to diastasis of the sutures
- Dense metaphyseal bands
- Vertebral bodies may show a bone-within-a-bone appearance due to repeated episodes

Further imaging
- None

Non-radiological investigations
- Blood lead levels
- Levels of haem precursors are lowered in early poisoning

Management The source of lead should be removed. Chelating agents may remove lead. In severe cases there is a poor outcome with neurological impairment.

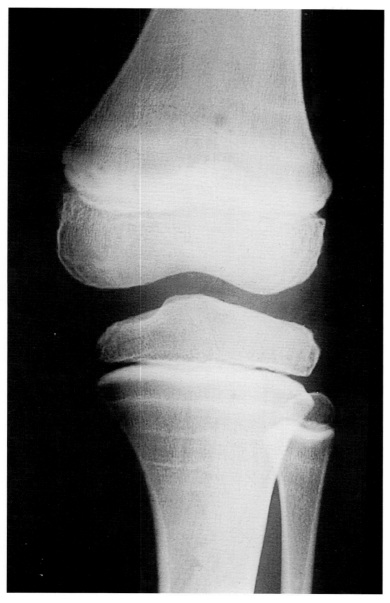

Fig 49.1 **AP knee.** Dense metaphyseal lines are seen in an otherwise normal joint.

50 **Lipoma**

Characteristics

- **Age range:** Generally seen in adults
- **Gender:** M = F (except spindle cell lipoma, 90% of which occur in males)
- **Incidence:** Very common
- **Pathology:** The tumour arises from normal fat and is multiple in at least 5%. On cross-section the lesion is a homogeneous pale to bright yellow colour. Histologically it consists of mature fat cells although pleomorphic and spindle cell lipomas do occur.

Clinical presentation Patients present with a soft, painless swelling which is well circumscribed. The shoulder girdle and proximal thigh are the most common sites. Eighty percent are of the subcutaneous type, although lipomas can occur at inter- and intramuscular sites, ✴ often mimicking soft tissue sarcomas. Spindle cell lipomas most commonly occur around the neck and shoulder.

Radiology

Description

- Larger tumours may be visible on plain films as a well-defined area of fat density
- US demonstrates a circumscribed ovoid lesion with striations similar to muscle

Further imaging

- On T1- and T2-weighted MR scans a well-defined lesion of high signal intensity is seen. The lesion should suppress completely on fat saturation sequences
- Imaging-guided biopsy may be necessary if there is clinical confusion

Non-radiological investigations

- None

Management Many lesions can be left alone. If necessary, simple surgical excision is curative. Deep lipomas may not have a capsule so wider resection can be required to achieve local control.

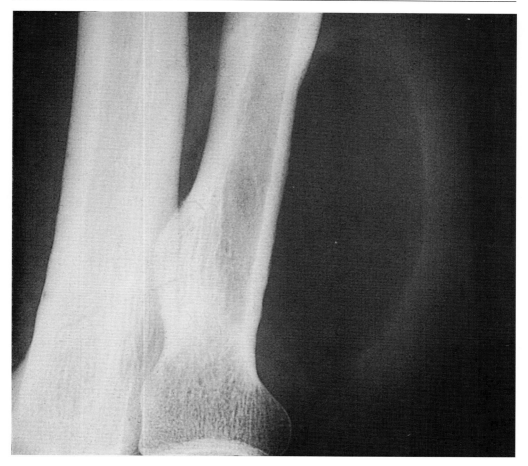

Fig 50.1 **AP elbow.** Adjacent to the bone there is a well-demarcated soft tissue lesion of fat density. There is no calcification.

51 **Liposarcoma**

Characteristics

- **Age range:** Most common in the fifth and sixth decades
- **Gender:** M = F
- **Incidence:** 12–18% of all malignant soft tissue tumours
- **Pathology:** Rarely it may arise from a preexisting benign lesion. May be well differentiated, myxoid, round cell or pleomorphic. The tumours tend to be well circumscribed and lobulate.

Clinical presentation
Patients may present with a large (10–15 cm) mass around the lower trunk or lower extremity. It should also be suspected if a fatty tumour continues to grow and becomes painful. Liposarcomas may be multiple and occur in unusual sites in one individual.

Radiology
Description
- Plain films may indicate the presence of a soft tissue mass, not necessarily of fat density
- Extensive calcification may be seen

Further imaging
- US shows a mixed echogenicity mass with disordered vascularity
- CT shows a mass of mixed fatty and solid attenuation, which may enhance on administration of intravenous contrast
- 🔑 Local staging with MR shows a high-signal lesion on T2 weighting, which does not suppress on fat-saturated sequences
- Imaging-guided biopsy
- CT thorax for distant staging

Non-radiological investigations
- Histology

Management
Low-grade lesions can be removed by wide excision, whereas high-grade tumours require radical resection or amputation. Radiation may be effective as an adjunct or for tumours in inaccessible sites.

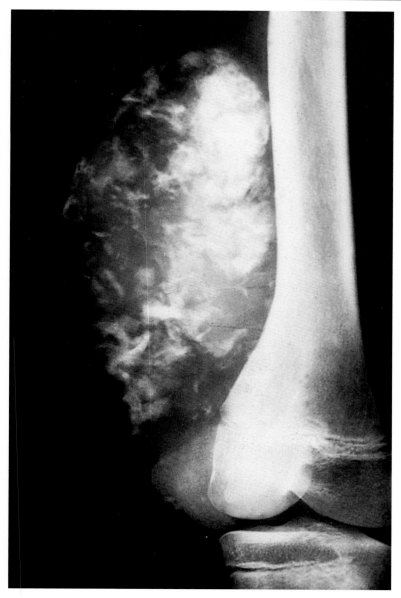

Fig 51.1 **AP knee.** There is a large soft tissue mass demonstrating a range of density from fat to markedly dystrophic calcification.

52 Lymphoma

Characteristics

- **Age range:** Most common in the third to fifth decades
- **Gender:** M:F = 2:1
- **Incidence:** 2–6% of all primary bone tumours in children
- **Pathology:** A round cell tumour of the reticuloendothelial system. Is usually a sign of disseminated disease but may rarely be a solitary lesion. Histology shows a marrow cell tumour with collections of abnormal lymphocytes.

Clinical presentation The incidence of bone involvement for known lymphomas is 5–15% in Hodgkin's and 25–40% in non-Hodgkin's disease. Patients generally present with a pathological fracture or pain in sites with abundant red cell marrow, i.e. flat bones, spine and the metaphyses of long bones.

Radiology

Description

- ☞ Diaphyseal or metaphyseal permeative lytic process with cortical destruction
- May be multifocal and sometimes is sclerotic
- Periosteal reaction is infrequently seen
- There may be an associated soft tissue mass

Further imaging

- Imaging-guided biopsy
- MR for local staging
- Chest, abdomen and pelvic CT and bone scan for distant staging

Non-radiological investigations

- Histology – differentiation between the types of lymphoma is critical for treatment and prognosis

Management A 5-year survival of 56% is achieved through combination chemotherapy (adriamycin, alkylating agents and steroids) and radiotherapy. The latter alone may be curative for solitary bone lymphoma. Surgery is limited to treating pathological fractures and, rarely, resection.

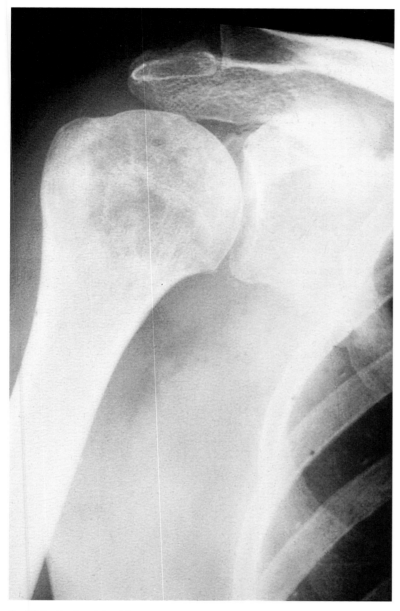

Fig 52.1 **AP shoulder.** There is permeative destruction in the humeral head.
Note, however, that there is some associated sclerosis.

53 **Madura foot**

Characteristics
- **Age range:** May present at any age
- **Gender:** M = F
- **Incidence:** Very rare
- **Pathology:** A chronic fungal infection due to maduromyces species. The organism enters through a small wound and inhabits the subcutaneous tissues and tendon sheaths in the foot. Bones and joints are affected by direct invasion. There may be secondary bacterial infection.

Clinical presentation Cutaneous sinuses are usually present, with a swollen and indurated foot.

Radiology
Description
- ☞ Chronic infection leads to mature periosteal reactions and sclerosis

- There is bizarre resorption and remodelling particularly affecting the metacarpals and phalanges
- Secondary infection leads to increasing destruction

Further imaging
- Imaging-guided biopsy may be appropriate

Non-radiological investigations
- Fungus is identified in discharge or biopsy

Management Is generally unsatisfactory. IV amphotericin B is used, although of high toxicity. The necrotic tissue must be widely excised and amputation may be necessary.

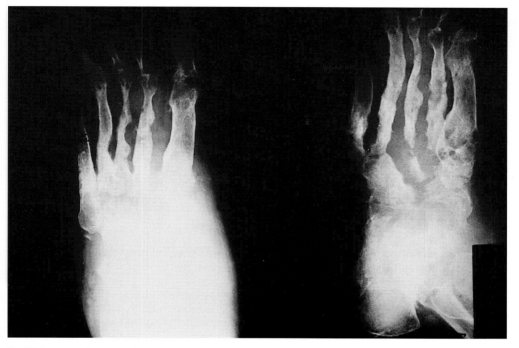

Fig 53.1 **DP and oblique foot.** There is a bizarre combination of bony sclerosis, mature periosteal reaction and bone destruction.

54 **Malignant fibrous histiocytoma (MFH)**

Characteristics
- **Age range:** Peak incidence is in the sixth decade but the age range is wide
- **Gender:** M:F = 3:2
- **Incidence:** 20–30% of all soft tissue sarcomas, 5% of bone sarcomas
- **Pathology:** MFH may affect bone or soft tissues. It is a fibrous tumour containing histiocytes and giant cells, which may be of storiform (commonest), myxoid, giant cell or inflammatory type.

Clinical presentation It is most common in the lower limb and lesions may be solitary or multifocal. 🔔 Extensive haemorrhage and necrosis lead to pain and swelling, which may lead to an erroneous clinical diagnosis of haematoma. The bone type occurs in abnormal bone, particularly at sites of old infarcts or other disease.

Radiology
Description
- 🔑 Permeative osteolytic lesion

- Usually in the metaphysis of long bones
- Rarely periosteal reaction unless a pathological fracture is present
- Presence of cortical destruction may indicate a soft tissue mass

Further imaging
- Imaging-guided biopsy
- MRI for local staging
- Chest CT and bone scan for distant staging

Non-radiological investigations
- Histology

Management Five-year survival is 50% and achieved through radical resection or amputation. Adjuvant chemotherapy is given and inaccessible tumours may require radiotherapy. Soft tissue myxoid lesions have a more favourable prognosis.

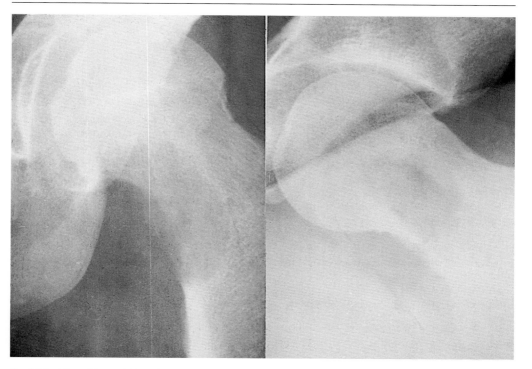

Fig 54.1 **AP and lateral hip.** There is a destructive, purely lytic lesion in the femoral neck.

55 Marfan's syndrome

Characteristics
- **Age range:** Infancy to adulthood
- **Gender:** M=F
- **Incidence:** Uncommon
- **Pathology:** Autosomal dominant. There is an abnormality of the fibrillin gene.

Clinical presentation The patients are tall with long arms and legs; the arm span exceeds the height. There is pectus excavatum, superior lens dislocation, a high-arched palate, aortic incompetence and an increased incidence of aortic dissection 🔔 . Joint laxity can lead to flat feet, patella and shoulder dislocations. There is an increased incidence of spondylolisthesis, scoliosis and SUFE.

Radiology
Description
- 🔑 Overtubulated bones, particularly in hands and feet – arachnodactyly
- Pes planus, hallux valgus, talipes, long great toe
- Scoliosis
- Sternal deformities
- Dural ectasia leads to posterior vertebral scalloping, increased interpediculate distance and large sacral foraminae
- Lax joints result in premature OA and recurrent dislocations
- Large mandible and a high, arched bony palate seen on SXR

Further imaging
- CXR and chest CT/MRI may be indicated for the assessment of cardiovascular complications such as dissecting thoracic aneurysm

Non-radiological investigations
- None

Management Mild to moderate scolioses are braced while severe, rigid curves should be considered for fusion.

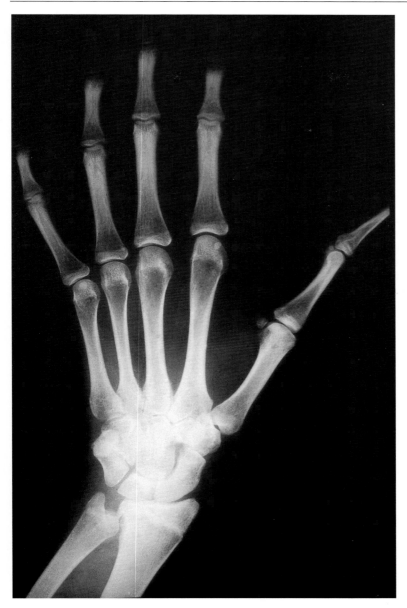

Fig 55.1 **DP hand.** Overtubulation (arachnodactyly) is seen in the long bones.

56 **Melorheostosis**

Characteristics
- **Age range:** May present at any age but commonly in childhood
- **Gender:** M = F
- **Incidence:** Rare
- **Pathology:** Dense cortical bone with soft tissue fibrosis. Distribution is along dermatomes.

Clinical presentation There are soft tissue contractures, often with severe fixed joint deformities and dislocations. The soft tissues are 'woody' with puckering of the skin and deep fascia. It is generally painless in children and painful in adults. Limb lengths are frequently unequal.

Radiology
Description
- Diaphyseal cortical thickening affects more than one bone of a single limb (usually lower)
- Smooth flowing hyperostosis likened to dripping candle wax, from proximal end of bone extending distally
- May cross a joint and distribution follows sclerotomes of individual spinal nerves

Further imaging
- None

Non-radiological investigations
- None

Management It often requires radical surgical soft tissue releases and long-term bracing during growth. The patient may require osteotomies and recurrent deformity with further growth is common. Amputation may be necessary.

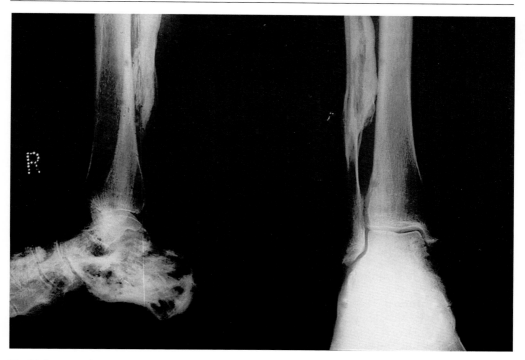

Fig 56.1 **AP and lateral ankle.** There is extensive cortical and periosteal thickening. Note the 'flowing candle wax' appearance in the fibula.

57 Meniscal tear

Characteristics
- **Age range:** Young adults, with a further peak in middle age
- **Gender:** M > F due to sporting activity
- **Incidence:** Very common
- **Pathology:** The menisci are critical for load distribution, shock absorption, joint stability, lubrication, articular cartilage nutrition and proprioception. Traumatic tears occur in young adults and may be vertical longitudinal (75%), oblique, transverse medial or horizontal. Degenerate tears occur in patients over the age of 40, often with minimal trauma.

Clinical presentation The young adult often presents after sustaining a twisting injury to a flexed knee. There is pain and delayed swelling and the knee may be locked. The joint line is tender and McMurray's test may be positive. In long-standing cases the quadriceps may be wasted. The medial meniscus is more commonly injured than the lateral and there may be associated ligamentous injuries. The older patient with a degenerate tear complains of pain, swelling, clicking, giving way and sometimes locking.

Radiology
Description
- Plain films may show an effusion

Further imaging
- ☞ MR demonstrates a line of high signal which reaches a free meniscal surface
- Complex tears show multiple, stellate signal changes
- An associated meniscal cyst may be shown on MR or US

Non-radiological investigations
- None

Management For the acutely injured knee, treatment includes analgesia, ice and elevation. If the knee remains locked or symptoms persist, arthroscopy is indicated. Physiotherapy can relieve the symptoms of a degenerate tear and maintain range of movement and quadriceps strength. Asymptomatic meniscal tears do not require treatment. Arthroscopic treatment options include partial meniscectomy, total meniscectomy and meniscal repair. The aim is to preserve the meniscus and meniscal repair is generally reserved for the young patient with an acute vertical tear of greater than 1.5 cm in length into the peripheral third which has a blood supply. The inner two-thirds is avascular, gaining its nutrition from the synovial fluid, and is not suitable for repair.

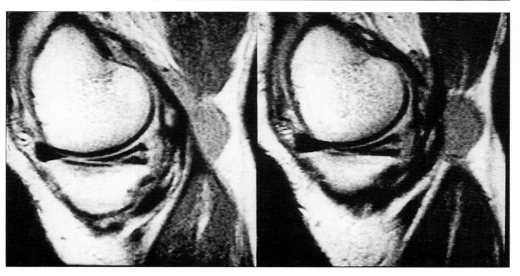

Fig 57.1 **T2-weighted sagittal MR of the knee.** An oblique line of high signal comes into contact with the inferior surface of the posterior horn of the medial meniscus.

58 Metaphyseal dysplasia (type Schmid)

Characteristics
- **Age range:** Presents in infancy
- **Gender:** M = F
- **Incidence:** Very rare
- **Pathology:** Autosomal dominant inheritance of a metaphyseal chondrodysplasia.

Clinical presentation
Patients are of short stature with short limbs. They have bowed limbs and a waddling gait. Shortness increases with age. The main differential diagnosis is rickets.

Radiology
Description
- There is mild splaying and irregularity of the metaphyses, most marked at the knees

- Enlarged capital femoral epiphyses, coxa vara and femoral bowing
- Ribs are invariably dense and splayed
- Bone density is normal

Further imaging
- None

Non-radiological investigations
- None

Management
Limb lengthening procedures may be necessary. Premature osteoarthritis may also require treatment.

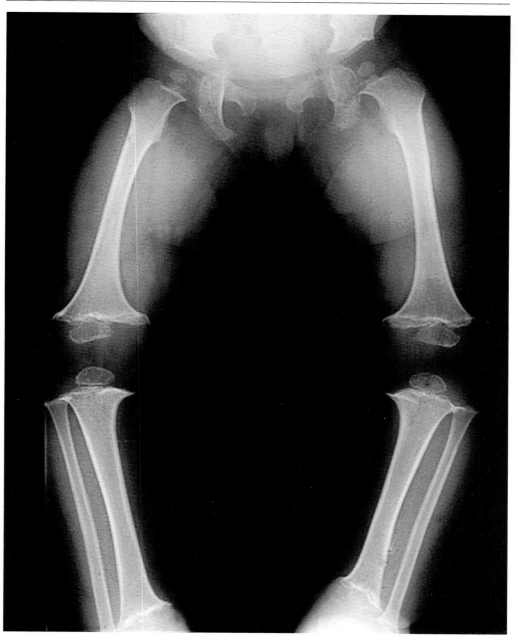

Fig 58.1 **AP lower limbs.** Note the splayed metaphyses in the presence of normal bone density and a normal provisional zone of calcification.

59 **Metastases**

Characteristics
- **Age range:** Most common from the fifth decade onwards
- **Gender:** M = F
- **Incidence:** Extremely common, series suggest 15–100 times the incidence of primary skeletal neoplasms
- **Pathology:** Probably due to venous tumour emboli. Bone metastases are most common from carcinoma of the lung, breast, prostate, kidney and thyroid.

Clinical presentation Patients may present with bone pain or a pathological fracture, with or without a known primary. They may present with symptoms from associated soft tissue metastases or lesions may be discovered by staging. Many lesions are solitary at presentation.

Radiology
Description
- ⚷ Lesions predominate in red marrow-containing parts of the skeleton, i.e. skull, spine, ribs and pelvis
- Rare beyond knees and elbows
- Lytic if there is no reactive bone formation
- Wide zone of transition
- Pathological fracture is common
- Does not cross joints or disc spaces
- Renal and thyroid carcinomas produce expansile lesions
- Breast and prostate carcinomas produce sclerotic lesions which may be extensive
- Sclerosis and periosteal reaction are also seen in pelvic adenocarcinoma primaries

Further imaging
- Bone scan to define the extent of disease, may show multiple areas of increased uptake or a 'superscan'
- CXR, mammogram, US, CT or MRI to find primary
- Imaging-guided biopsy if unknown primary

Non-radiological investigations
- Cytology
- Histology
- Serum tumour markers may help identify a primary

Management Identify the site of the primary if not already known. Chemotherapy or radiotherapy depending on the histology; fixation of pathological fractures.

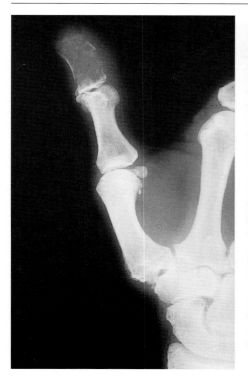

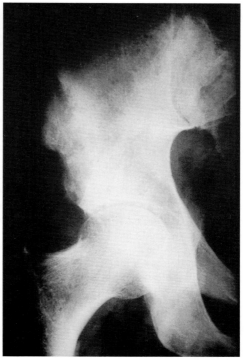

Fig 59.1 **Lateral thumb.** There is a lytic lesion in the terminal phalanx with a pathological fracture. This was from a bronchial primary, which is the carcinoma most commonly metastasizing to the periphery.

Fig 59.2 **AP hip.** There is generalized patchy increase in bone density from sclerotic prostatic metastases.

60 Morquio's disease (mucopolysaccharidosis IV)

Characteristics
- **Age range:** Childhood
- **Gender:** M = F
- **Incidence:** Very rare
- **Pathology:** ☞ Deficiency of galactosamine-6-sulphatase leading to defective degradation of keratin sulphate. Autosomal recessive.

Clinical presentation Development normal for first 1–2 years. Thereafter the child becomes dwarfed, deaf and lax jointed, leading to progressive genu valgum. There is a moderate kyphosis and short neck and a marked manubriosternal angle is characteristic. Aortic regurgitation may be present. The face and intelligence are normal.

Radiology
Description
- Platyspondyly
- Central anterior vertebral beak
- ☀ Hypoplastic odontoid peg leads to C1/2 instability
- Wide interpediculate distance

- Thoracolumbar scoliosis
- Flared iliac wings and constricted iliac bodies produce a 'goblet'-shaped pelvis
- Delayed ossification of the capital femoral epiphysis produces coxa valga
- Delayed ossification of the lateral proximal tibial epiphysis produces a sloping tibial plateau
- Short forearms with carpal anomalies
- Variable rib anomalies
- Premature OA

Further imaging
- None

Non-radiological investigations
- None

Management No specific treatment. Surgery is often required for genu valgum (corrective osteotomy), coxa valga and subluxation of the hips (femoral or acetabular osteotomy generally only required if unilateral) and atlantoaxial instability (occipitocervical fusion).

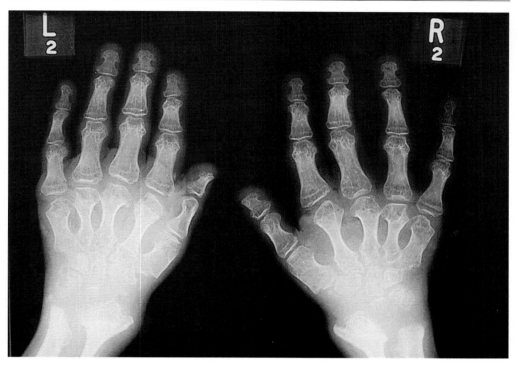

Fig 60.1 **DP hand.** Gross undertubulation of the bones is seen. There is splaying of the metaphysis, particularly at the distal radius. Some central tapering of the metacarpals is demonstrated.

61 Myeloma

Characteristics

- **Age range:** Most common in the fifth and sixth decades; 98% of patients are over the age of 40
- **Gender:** M:F = 2:1
- **Incidence:** Most common primary bone neoplasm in adults
- **Pathology:** Believed to arise from the plasma cells of bone marrow. Tumours are found in red marrow areas, the trunk and proximal axial skeleton. Histology reveals sheets of plasmacytes with large, eccentric nuclei. Lesions are multiple at presentation.

Clinical presentation Patients present with weakness, bone pain and pathological fractures. Patients may also present with signs and symptoms related to bone marrow suppression, hypercalcaemia and renal failure. Infection and renal failure are the most common causes of death and either is a poor prognosticator.

Radiology
Description
- Skeletal survey defines the pattern of disease
- Generalized osteopenia
- ☞ A permeative lytic pattern in the long bones
- Multiple 'punched out' cortical deposits may produce scalloping and are most common in the long bones and skull
- Extremely rarely produces sclerotic lesions

Further imaging
- ☀ Isotope scanning may miss 25–50% of lesions

Non-radiological investigations
- Bence Jones proteins in the urine
- Monoclonal paraprotein on serum electrophoresis
- Raised ESR and anaemia

Management Radiotherapy and chemotherapy may relieve pain from bone lesions. Pathological fractures may be internally fixed and cavities filled with methylmethacrylate cement.

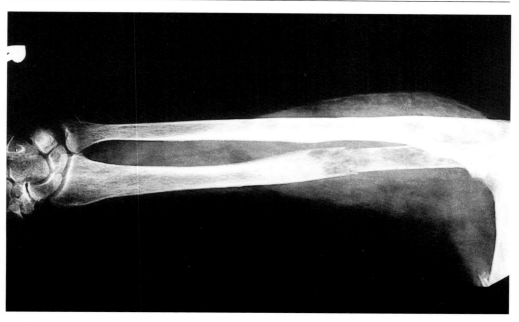

Fig 61.1 **AP forearm.** There is a permeative, lytic, destructive lesion in the proximal shaft of the radius with a pathological fracture.

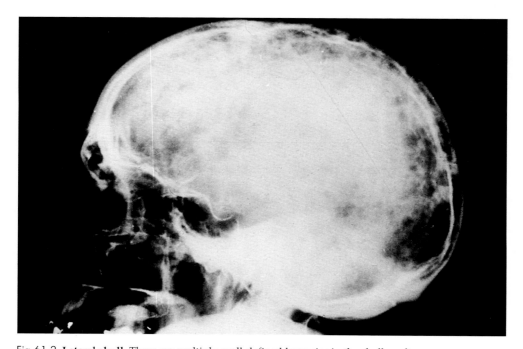

Fig 61.2 **Lateral skull.** There are multiple, well-defined lucencies in the skull vault.

62 Neurofibromatosis (NF)

Characteristics
- **Age range:** Any age
- **Gender:** M = F
- **Incidence:** 1 in 3000 births
- **Pathology:** Autosomal dominant inheritance with variable penetrance. A benign tumour of fibrous and neural elements. Macroscopically it is a pale fibrous lesion with nerve elements running into and through the tumour. Microscopically there are fibrillar and cellular components arranged in a wavy pattern (Schwann cells with collagen fibrils and myxoid material). It generally affects peripheral nerves, although the autonomic and central nervous systems are involved. It may arise directly in bone, when there is more of a cystic component.

Clinical presentation Lesions arising from a peripheral nerve may be obvious, though often it is seen as a nodule in the skin or subcutaneous tissue. May be solitary or multiple. Type I – multiple NF (von Recklinghausen's disease). There are numerous skin nodules and café-au-lait spots. It may be associated with skeletal abnormalities such as scoliosis, pseudarthrosis or limb hypertrophy. Malignant transformation of nerve sheath tumours occurs in 5–10% of cases. Type II – bilateral acoustic neuromas. Unlikely to exhibit cutaneous signs.

Radiology
Description
- Vertebral anomalies lead to kyphoscoliosis

- Posterior scalloping of vertebral bodies and hypoplastic pedicles due to dural ectasia
- Neurofibromas may cause enlargement of neural exit foraminae
- Ribbon ribs with inferior notching
- ⟁ Pseudarthroses
- Cortical erosion from soft tissue neurofibromas
- Poorly developed sphenoid bone with an 'empty orbit' due to enlarged optic foramen
- Widened internal auditory meati due to neuromas
- Lytic calvarial lesions, particularly adjacent to the lambdoid suture

Further imaging
- CT/MR for associated gliomas, meningiomas and neuromas, as well as nerve sheath tumours

Non-radiological investigations
- None

Management Treatment is only required if pain or paraesthesia becomes troublesome or if a tumour becomes very large or malignant change is suspected. Local excision is performed en bloc if an unimportant nerve or intracapsular shelling is performed if nerve damage is not acceptable. Malignancy is treated as appropriate.

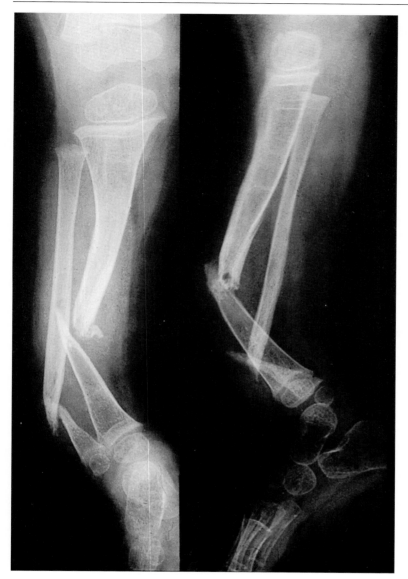

Fig 62.1 **AP and lateral lower leg.** Pseudarthroses are noted in the tibia and fibula. Note the tapered ends of the bones.

63 Neuropathic joint (Charcot joint)

Characteristics

- **Age range:** Depends on the underlying pathology but characteristically middle age and elderly
- **Gender:** M = F
- **Incidence:** Uncommon
- **Pathology:** Loss of pain sensation and proprioception in the joint leads to repeated trauma and destruction. This is commonly due to diabetes; rare cases due to tabes dorsalis still present. In the shoulder, the condition is due most commonly to syringomyelia. It can occur in any condition producing a sensory neuropathy but in 20% no neuropathy is found.

Clinical presentation The patient may present with restriction of movement, swelling or deformity as the joint is usually painless. A Charcot shoulder, however, may present with pain.

Radiology

Description

- Gross destruction of the joint
- Bony debris within the joint capsule
- ☞ Increased or normal bone density as the patient continues to use the affected joint

Further imaging

- MR of the cervical or lumbar spine to evaluate a potential underlying cause

Non-radiological investigations

- Appropriate to identifying the underlying cause, e.g. fasting glucose, syphilis serology

Management Treatment of the underlying cause is indicated with mechanical reconstruction or replacement as necessary.

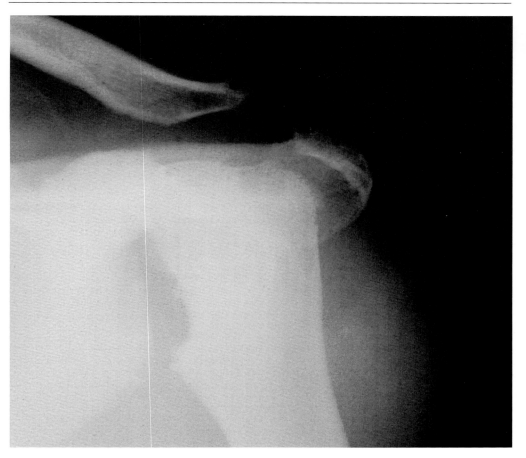

Fig 63.1 **AP shoulder.** There is destruction of all compartments of the joint. The bone density is increased and calcified debris can just be seen in a large effusion.

64 **Non-accidental injury**

Characteristics
- **Age range:** Children, predominantly infants and toddlers
- **Gender:** M = F
- **Incidence:** Estimated as the cause for 5–10% of injuries seen in children in US accident and emergency departments. Probably accounts for thousands of deaths each year.
- **Pathology:** Risk factors for child abuse include: mother aged less than 30, unwanted pregnancy, marital stress, lower social groups. Mechanisms of injury include twisting, sudden pulls and shaking.

Clinical presentation The parents give a history often inconsistent with the severity of the injuries; presentation may be late after the injury. The accompanying adult may not be a parent and there may be unexplained fractures or injuries of differing ages. Clinical indications may be ruptured tongue frenulum, conjunctival haemorrhages and cigarette burns.

Radiology
Description
- Multiple fractures of varying age and distribution
- Metaphyseal fragmentation and there may be a large 'bucket handle' fragment which is pathognomonic and produced by a twisting force
- Epiphyseal separation
- Spiral fractures of long bones in a non-ambulant child suggesting a rotatory force
- Periosteal reaction from subperiosteal haemorrhage
- Marked callus formation and cortical thickening which extends to the epiphyseal plate
- Fractures in suspicious sites such as posterior ribs, scapula, sternum and lateral clavicle
- Skull fractures, particularly occipital

Further imaging
- Head CT for intracranial haemorrhage
- Abdominal US/CT for visceral damage
- Head MRI may demonstrate haemorrhage of different ages and is sensitive for shearing injuries and changes due to hypoxia

Non-radiological investigations
- These may be indicated to exclude underlying skeletal or connective tissue abnormality

Management Consider the possibility of NAI in all suspicious or odd fractures in a child. Treat the fracture or injuries as clinically indicated and involve a senior paediatrician immediately.

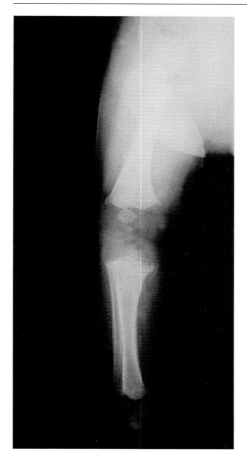

Fig 64.1 **AP leg.** There are metaphyseal fractures of the distal femur and proximal tibia, with femoral periosteal reaction.

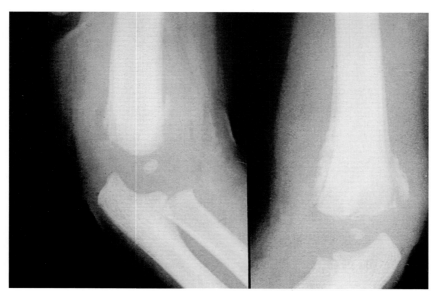

Fig 64.2 **AP and lateral elbow.** There is extensive periosteal reaction associated with metaphyseal fractures.

65 Non-ossifying fibroma/fibrous cortical defect

Characteristics
- **Age range:** Children and adolescents
- **Gender:** M > F
- **Incidence:** Common
- **Pathology:** A developmental defect where fibrous tissue is present in bone. Histologically, fibrous tissue is interspersed with occasional giant cells. There is no risk of malignant transformation.

Clinical presentation Usually an incidental finding as the lesion itself is asymptomatic. It occurs most frequently around the knee and pathological fractures can occur in larger lesions.

Radiology
Description
- ⚷ The fibrous cortical defect is a lucent, metaphyseal lesion less than 3 cm

- Narrow zone of transition
- Larger, multilocular lesions are termed non-ossifying fibroma

Further imaging
- None

Non-radiological investigations
- None

Management Most lesions spontaneously sclerose and remodel. Pathological fracture should be allowed to heal naturally. Larger defects may require curettage which is curative. Bone graft is not required. 🔔 Multiple lesions may be familial and bilateral lesions are associated with neurofibromatosis.

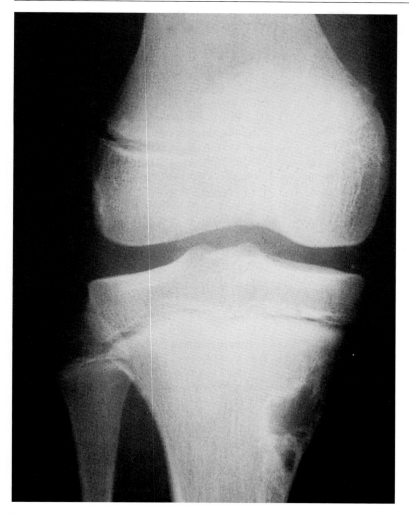

Fig 65.1 **AP knee.** There is a well-defined lucent cortical lesion which is multiloculate and has sclerotic margins.

66 Ollier's disease (enchondromatosis) and Mafucci's syndrome

Characteristics
- **Age range:** Presents at all ages
- **Gender:** M > F
- **Incidence:** Common (probably underreported)
- **Pathology:** A non-hereditary generalized disorder of endochondral bone formation. Cartilaginous rests fail to ossify and continue to grow within the metaphysis. Malignant change occurs in up to 30%.

Clinical presentation There is limb length discrepancy and lumps on the hands or feet. Increasing pain in adulthood may indicate malignant transformation. An associated arteriovenous malformation (Mafucci's syndrome) may be obvious. Mafucci's has a later presentation with a higher incidence of malignancy.

Radiology
Description
- ⚷ Multiple well-defined, expansile lesions containing punctate calcification are seen

- Small bones of the hand are predominantly affected
- Madelung deformity may occur
- Distribution is markedly asymmetrical
- Modelling abnormalities are seen
- Pathological fractures occur
- ☀ Enlargement and loss of definition suggest malignant change
- Small round opacities in the soft tissues indicate an associated AVM

Further imaging
- MR and imaging-guided biopsy if malignancy is suspected

Non-radiological investigations
- Histology

Management Surgery may be performed for cosmetic reasons, to treat pathological fractures or mechanical problems. Treatment for malignant change as appropriate.

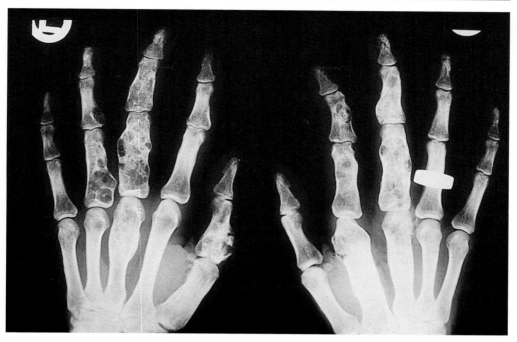

Fig 66.1 **DP both hands.** Multiple expansile, well-defined lesions are seen in several bones of both hands. These demonstrate small calcific densities within them.

67 Osteoarthritis

Characteristics
- **Age range:** Middle age to elderly
- **Gender:** M = F
- **Incidence:** Very common
- **Pathology:** Destruction and loss of hyaline articular cartilage. Initially there is an increase in water content, then loss of proteoglycans with secondary damage to chondrocytes and release of destructive cellular enzymes. It may be primary, where there is a strong genetic predisposition, or secondary due to previous insult to the articular cartilage.

Clinical presentation Pain and stiffness in affected joints, although it may be asymptomatic. Joints can be swollen and there is often crepitus on movement. Fixed deformities can occur. Heberden's nodes, at the distal interphalangeal joints, occur in postmenopausal women.

Radiology
Description
- ☞ Asymmetrical joint space loss in weight-bearing areas
- Non-weight bearing areas develop osteophytes
- Subchondral sclerosis
- Collapse of subarticular cysts leads to an appearance of erosions
- Bone density is preserved

Further imaging
- None

Non-radiological investigations
- None

Management Pain and disability are relieved by a combination of analgesia (non-steroidal antiinflammatories and paracetamol) and physiotherapy which maintains range of movement and muscle strength. Weight loss can help knee arthritis but is much less effective for the hip. Surgery may eventually be indicated – osteotomy, replacement arthroplasty, interposition arthroplasty, excision arthroplasty or arthrodesis.

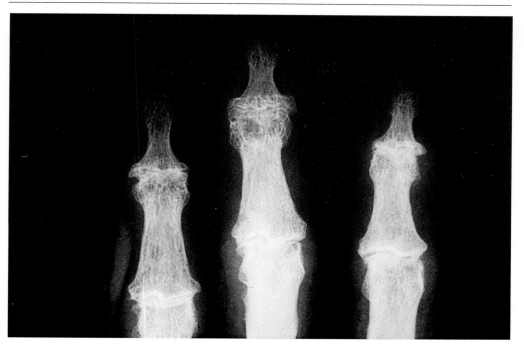

Fig 67.1 **DP fingers.** There is a combination of marked, asymmetrical joint space loss, with subchondral cysts and osteophyte formation.

68 **Osteoblastoma**

Characteristics
- **Age range:** Most often seen between 6 and 30 years
- **Gender:** M:F = 2:1
- **Incidence:** Rare, 3% of benign bone tumours
- **Pathology:** The tumour is very similar to an osteoid osteoma but larger (up to 10 cm) and more cellular. It is well circumscribed and has a fleshy appearance. Often highly vascular with areas of gritty osteoid formation. 🔔 Very rarely, malignant change can occur.

Clinical presentation Presenting features are pain (less than in osteoid osteoma) and local muscle spasm. Lesions in the spine and skull account for 50% of cases.

Radiology
Description
- 🔑 Lesions resemble osteoid osteoma, but larger

- A central lucent area of variable size is identified
- Significant reactive sclerosis is seen

Further imaging
- Markedly increased uptake on bone scan
- CT and MR may define the lesion more accurately
- Imaging-guided biopsy

Non-radiological investigations
- None

Management Excision and bone grafting. Often excision is incomplete due to the location and then local recurrence is common. Radiotherapy may be required for repeated recurrence.

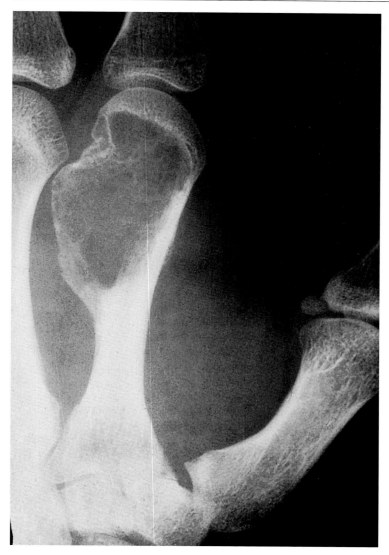

Fig 68.1 **DP hand.** A relatively well-defined expansile lesion which is entirely lytic is seen in the index finger metacarpal.

69 Osteochondral defect

Characteristics
- **Age range:** Adolescents and young adults
- **Gender:** M = F
- **Incidence:** Common
- **Pathology:** A defect of bone and overlying cartilage. May either be secondary to osteochondritis dissecans (OCD) or a single episode of trauma. Most commonly affects the medial femoral condyle but may also affect the talus, capitellum and first metatarsal head.

Clinical presentation Pain and swelling. The joint may be locked due to a loose osteochondral fragment. If secondary to OCD, there may be a preceding history of pain and discomfort.

Radiology
Description
- ☞ A well-defined corticated ovoid bony fragment is surrounded by lucency
- The underlying bone appears normal
- The fragment may become detached and be seen as a large loose body in the joint

Further imaging
- MRI is necessary to evaluate the cartilage cover of the lesion
- MR arthrography may show contrast tracking under the flap or an effusion may give a similar appearance
- In acute lesions oedema is seen on MR in local bone

Non-radiological investigations
- None

Management If the injury is acute, the joint is locked or a loose fragment can be seen on the radiograph, then surgery is indicated. Arthroscopy is performed and, if possible, the fresh loose fragment is replaced in the defect and held with tapered screws, which are buried beneath the articular cartilage. Sclerotic, avascular loose fragments are generally removed and the defect is either curetted or drilled to promote fibrocartilage growth.

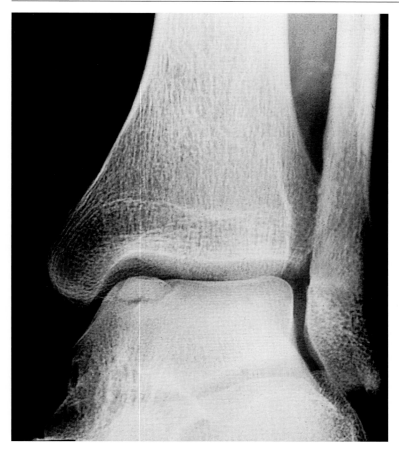

Fig 69.1 **AP ankle.** A well-defined osteochondral lesion is identified in the medial aspect of the talar dome. A zone of lucency surrounds this.

70 **Osteochondritis**

Characteristics
- **Age range:** Seen mostly in adolescence
- **Gender:** M > F
- **Incidence:** Common
- **Pathology:** A group of conditions where there is fragmentation or separation of a small segment of bone and articular cartilage. It shows many of the features of avascular necrosis and may be caused by a single episode of trauma or repeated stress. There are no signs of inflammation and pathological changes are the same as in other forms of bone necrosis, i.e. bone death, fragmentation and new bone formation. Syndromes consist of crushing, splitting or pulling types.

Clinical presentation The patient presents with pain, swelling and often a joint effusion. Specific syndromes are associated with disease at certain sites – Kienbock's disease of the lunate, Freiburg's disease of the second metatarsal head and Kohler's disease of the navicular are all crushing types. In the splitting form (osteochondritis dissecans) the joint may become locked if the necrotic fragment becomes detached, which happens most commonly in the knee. Pulling osteochondritis (or traction apophysitis) classically affects the tibial tuberosity (Osgood–Schlatter's disease) and the calcaneal apophysis (Sever's disease), and they do not produce bone necrosis. They are locally painful and tender, especially after activity.

Radiology
Description
- Osteochondritis dissecans in the knee classically affects the internal side of the medial femoral condyle
- A smooth corticated ovoid fragment is seen best on the tunnel view
- May become loose and lie in the joint
- ☞ At other sites collapse and sclerosis of the epiphysis or subarticular bone are seen
- Soft tissue swelling may be associated

Further imaging
- Oedematous changes are seen on MRI
- Bone scan is variably positive

Non-radiological investigations
- None

Management Treatment involves analgesia, rest and load reduction. Pulling osteochondritis may require a period of splint immobilization if pain is severe. Physiotherapy is useful for symptomatic relief and maintenance of muscle strength. If a fragment becomes detached then surgery is indicated for removal or fixation of the fragment (if not sclerotic or necrotic). Crushing osteochondritis may be amenable to a vascularized graft or osteotomy/ shortening if there is a disparity in bone length.

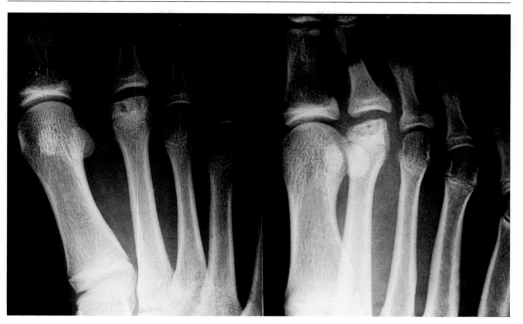

Fig 70.1 **DP foot.** Mixed sclerosis and lysis of the second metatarsal head is seen. There is also flattening. This is an example of Freiburg's disease.

71 **Osteochondroma (cartilage capped exostosis)**

Characteristics
- **Age range:** Seen most frequently in the first to third decades
- **Gender:** M = F
- **Incidence:** Most common benign bone lesion
- **Pathology:** It starts as an overgrowth of cartilage at the edge of the physeal plate, then endochondral ossification occurs forming a bony protuberance covered by a cartilage cap. It is sessile or pedunculated, characteristically in a long bone.

Clinical presentation Patients present with a lump which may be painful due to local bursitis, mechanical irritation of overlying tissues or pathological fracture. The mass continues to grow until skeletal maturity is reached. Pain or increased growth in an adult raises the possibility of malignant change (1% if solitary), which is more common in proximal than distal lesions.

Radiology
Description
- A bony protuberance is seen at the physeal scar which characteristically points away from the joint
- Calcification can be seen in the overlying cartilage cap
- ☞ Normal trabeculations are seen extending into the base of the lesion

Further imaging
- ☀ US or MR shows the thickness of the cartilage cap; the larger the cap, the higher the likelihood of malignant change

Non-radiological investigations
- Histology

Management Any tumour causing symptoms, or increasing in size in an adult, should be excised. Generally, those tumours arising from the axial skeleton, shoulder or pelvic girdle should also be excised.

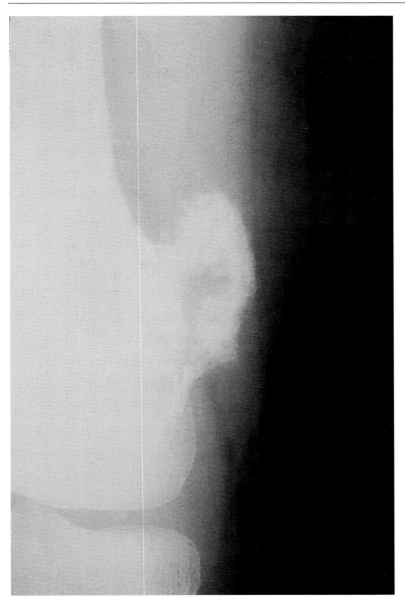

Fig 71.1 **AP knee.** There is an exostosis from the distal femoral metaphysis. Note that trabeculations are seen running into the base of the lesion. There is early calcification of the cartilage cap.

72 Osteogenesis imperfecta

Characteristics

- **Age range:** Presents from birth to adolescence
- **Gender:** M = F
- **Incidence:** 1 in 28 500 live births
- **Pathology:** There are four major subgroups but all show defective synthesis of type II collagen (α1 and α2 chains): Type I – mild, Type II – lethal at birth, Type III – severe deforming, and Type IV – moderately severe. May be autosomal recessive or dominant. The bone is immature and disorganized without a normal cortex.

Clinical presentation There are multiple fractures and subsequent bony deformities. There is associated dwarfing, bossed frontal bones and hypermobile joints; 60% have blue or transparent sclerae, 50% have dentinogenesis imperfecta and 50% become deaf. Fractures are much less common after adolescence.

Radiology
Description
- Generalized profound osteopenia

- ☞ Long bones are thin with bowing deformities and evidence of multiple fractures
- Exuberant callus formation
- Dislocations and pseudarthroses may develop
- Persistent Wormian bones
- Biconcave vertebral bodies with Schmorl's nodes
- Platybasia

Further imaging
- May be diagnosed by ultrasound antenatally if there is a poorly developed skeleton and intrauterine fractures

Non-radiological investigations
- None

Management The aim is to prevent injury by careful nursing of infants. Fractures are splinted to correct deformity. Intramedullary rods (often elongating to accommodate growth) may be used in long bones. Osteotomies may be necessary to correct deformities.

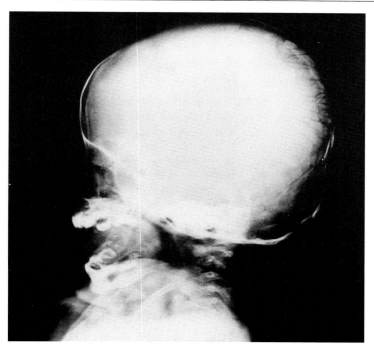

Fig 72.1 **Lateral skull.** Multiple Wormian bones are present in the posterior part of the skull.

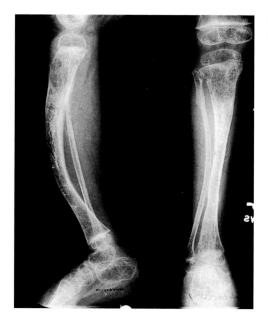

Fig 72.2 **AP and lateral lower leg.** There is profound osteopenia and evidence of multiple previous fractures.

73 Osteoid osteoma

Characteristics
- **Age range:** Half present between the ages of 10 and 20 years
- **Gender:** M:F = 2:1
- **Incidence:** Common, 12% of all benign bone tumours
- **Pathology:** Histologically there is a cherry-red nidus consisting of osteoblast-lined trabeculae and there may be prominent mineralization of the osteoid. Malignant change does not occur.

Clinical presentation Classically it is an extremely painful tumour, particularly at night. The pain is well localized to the site of the tumour and any bone can be affected although they are most often seen in the femur or tibia. Spinal lesions are also common. Typically the pain is abolished by salicylates. Osteoid osteoma can be difficult to diagnose as pain may precede radiological abnormality; secondary features such as limping, muscle wasting or scoliosis may then occur.

Radiology
Description
- There is a small lucency, the nidus, sometimes with a central dot of calcification
- Surrounding reactive sclerosis gives rise to a target appearance
- Excessive surrounding sclerosis may obscure the nidus
- When arising in a bone with little periosteum there may be no sclerosis

Further imaging
- Markedly increased uptake on bone scan
- CT is the method of choice for showing the nidus
- MR is non-specific and not recommended
- Imaging-guided biopsy or excision

Non-radiological investigations
- Histology

Management The nidus must be totally removed either at surgery or by CT guidance.

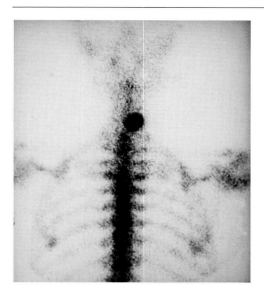

Fig 73.1 **Static bone scan.** A focus of high isotope uptake is seen in the left side of the lower cervical spine.

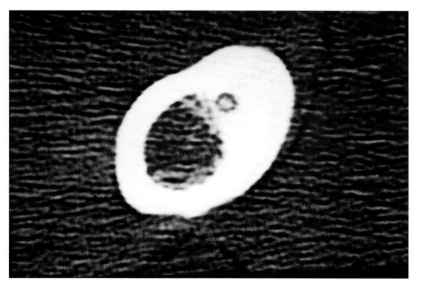

Fig 73.2 **CT femur.** The small lucent nidus is identified as a target lesion within an area of profound bony sclerosis.

74 Osteomalacia

Characteristics
- **Age range:** Adulthood
- **Gender:** M = F
- **Incidence:** Not uncommon
- **Pathology:** Generally due to a deficiency of vitamin D or its metabolism, e.g. nutritional deficiency, lack of sunlight, malabsorption, liver disease (decreased 25-hydroxylation) and renal disease (decreased 1α-hydroxylation). Normal bone matrix fails to mineralize and histologically there is excess osteoid.

Clinical presentation There is usually an insidious onset with proximal myopathy, bone pain and backache. The patient may develop a mild kyphosis due to vertebral collapse and Looser's zones may become pathological fractures.

Radiology
Description
- Overall the bone mineral density is reduced
- Looser's zones develop. These are short, lucent lines seen particularly at the lateral margin of the scapula and the medial femoral neck
- Transverse fractures may occur
- Vertebral collapse may be seen

Further imaging
- Looser's zones are hot on bone scanning

Non-radiological investigations
- Plasma calcium is normal or low
- Plasma phosphate is low
- Alkaline phosphatase is high
- Urinary calcium excretion is very low
- In vitamin D deficiency plasma 25-hydroxylated D is low

Management Treatment of the underlying cause is indicated. Generally large doses of calcium and vitamin D are given so the biochemistry needs careful monitoring during treatment.

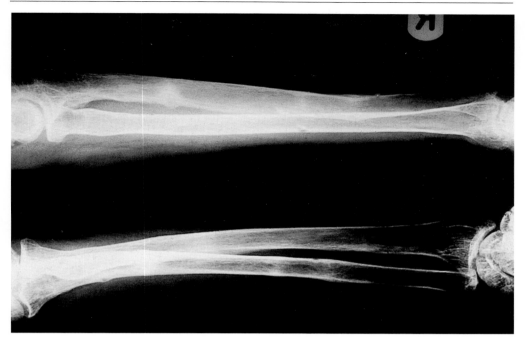

Fig 74.1 **AP and lateral forearm.** There is profound osteopenia. Multiple pseudofractures or Looser's zones are seen.

75 Osteopathia striata

Characteristics
- **Age range:** Any age
- **Gender:** M = F
- **Incidence:** Rare
- **Pathology:** Probably autosomal dominant inheritance

Clinical presentation An incidental finding of no significance.

Radiology
Description
- ☞ Dense longitudinal streaking of the metaphysis of long bones
- May extend into the epiphysis and metaphysis
- Occasionally also affects ilium and vertebral bodies

Further imaging
- Nil

Non-radiological investigations
- Nil

Management None, but the 'streaks' may mimic congenital rubella lesions 🔔.

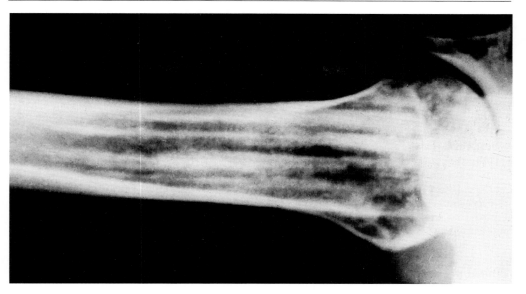

Fig 75.1 **Axial shoulder.** Long dense streaks extend parallel to the diaphysis.

76 Osteopetrosis (marble bone, Albers–Schonberg disease)

Characteristics
- **Age range:** Depending on the subtype, may present at any age from infancy
- **Gender:** M = F
- **Incidence:** Rare
- **Pathology:** There is a reduction in the normal marrow cells controlling osteoclastic activity. There are two forms: severe autosomal recessive and benign autosomal dominant. Bone formation is excessive but in the benign form it 'switches on and off'.

Clinical presentation The recessive form results in pancytopenia from marrow encroachment and the features of extramedullary haemopoiesis. Cranial nerve palsies, deafness and blindness can occur secondary to compression. ☀ Death may occur in early childhood. The benign form may be discovered as an incidental finding although pathological fractures, cranial nerve compression and osteomyelitis are relatively common.

Radiology
Description
- Generalized uniform increase in bone density
- Loss of trabeculation
- All bones and all parts of bone may be involved although rare in mandible
- ☀ 'Bone within bone' appearance
- Small paranasal sinuses and skull base foramina
- Shortening of long bones
- Pathological fractures
- Soft tissue calcification

Further imaging
- Head CT may be indicated to assess the skull foramina

Non-radiological investigations
- Full blood count

Management The severe form may be treated by bone marrow transplantation. Otherwise treatment is only indicated for complications.

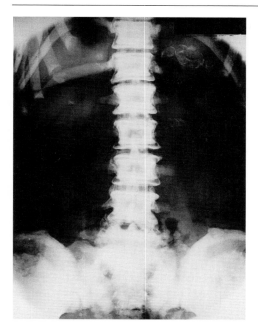

Fig 76.1 **AP spine.** Note the 'bone within bone'
appearance seen throughout the spine.

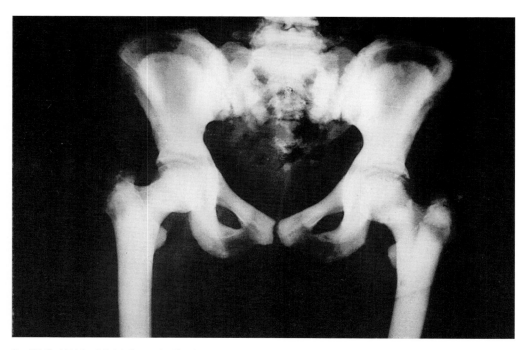

Fig 76.2 **AP hip.** Multiple markedly dense regions parallel the natural shape of the bone.

77 Osteopoikilosis

Characteristics
- **Age range:** Any age
- **Gender:** M = F
- **Incidence:** Rare
- **Pathology:** Autosomal dominant inheritance

Clinical presentation Usually an incidental finding but may be associated with cutaneous white spots – disseminated lenticular fibrosis.

Radiology
Description
- 🔑 Round or ovoid foci of bone sclerosis (2–10 mm)

- Located in metaphysis and epiphysis but not in diaphysis, so commonly concentrated around the joints
- Most commonly distributed around hip
- Small bones of hands and feet may also be involved

Further imaging
- None

Non-radiological investigations
- None

Management ☀ None needed, although it may need to be differentiated from diffuse sclerotic metastases.

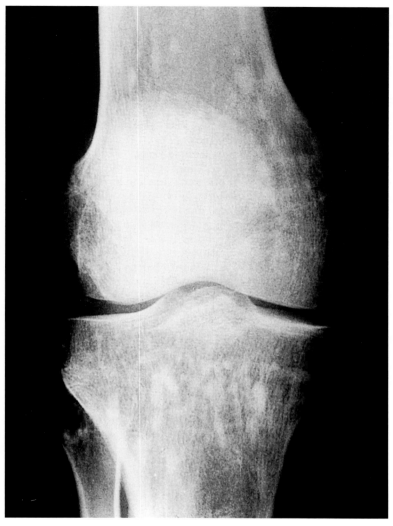

Fig 77.1 **AP knee.** Multiple dense ovoid lesions are seen scattered around the joint.

78 **Osteoporosis**

Characteristics
- **Age range:** Most often seen over 65 years
- **Gender:** Marked female preponderance
- **Incidence:** Extremely common; seen in one in three women over 65 years of age
- **Pathology:** Defined as reduced bone mass of normal composition. It is most commonly idiopathic in postmenopausal women who may lose up to 8% of their bone mass per year. Males over 60 years may lose up to 3%. It can be secondary to numerous disorders such as congenital abnormalities, endocrinopathy – particularly excess steroids – immobility, arthritis, infiltration by malignancy and drugs. May also be localized and transient, most often in the hip in pregnancy.

Clinical presentation Patients typically present with insufficiency fractures (fractures produced by normal activity or trivial injury), especially in the hip, spine and radius. Screening can be carried out by bone densitometry.

Radiology
Description
- 🔑 Diagnosis is made by reduced density at dual energy X-ray absorptiometry (DEXA)
- 🔔 Plain films are highly unreliable
- Calibrated CT is an accurate method of diagnosis
- Loss of bone density
- 'Pencilling' of the cortical margin
- Loss of random and horizontal trabecular pattern, leaving the vertical
- Wedging of the vertebrae with irregular endplates leads to loss of height and kyphosis
- Fractures may be difficult to see due to lack of medullary or cortical bone
- Skull sutures appear prominent

Further imaging
- Occult fractures may require isotope scanning or MR for diagnosis

Non-radiological investigations
- None

Management Diet, exercise and HRT may prevent osteoporosis from developing. Treatment is with calcitonin, diphosphonates and sodium fluoride.

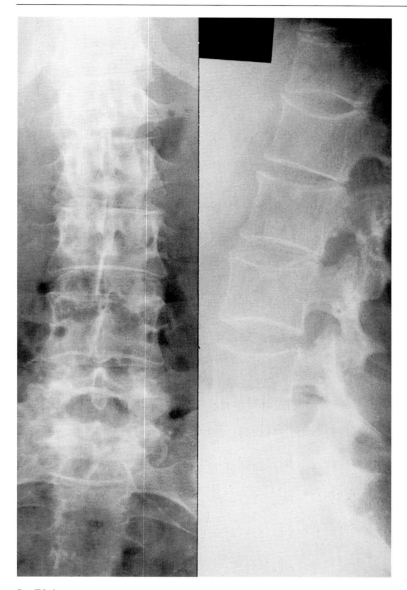

Fig 78.1 **AP and lateral spine.** There is profound loss of bone density but no
evidence of wedge fractures.

79 Osteosarcoma

Characteristics
- **Age range:** Peak incidence in the second and third decade, with a smaller peak in the elderly in association with Paget's disease
- **Gender:** M:F = 2:1
- **Incidence:** 4–5 cases per million per year, classic osteosarcoma constituting 72% of cases
- **Pathology:** A high-grade malignant spindle cell tumour with a typical microscopic appearance of osteoid arising from neoplastic cells which have a high alkaline phosphatase. The primary tumour is often very vascular, resulting in early haematogenous spread. Histologically it may be chondroblastic, osteoblastic or telangiectatic.

Clinical presentation The patient presents with pain (often worse at night), swelling or occasionally pathological fracture. It arises in the metaphysis of long bones; 75% occur around the knee, 9% in the proximal humerus. The axial skeleton is rarely affected. Examination shows a firm, tender, soft tissue mass fixed to the underlying bone. Systemic symptoms are rare. Lung metastases are common.

Radiology
Description
- An aggressive metaphyseal lesion with a wide zone of transition
- ☛ Tumour bone formation is identified with matrix mineralization and soft tissue new bone formation
- There may be a soft tissue mass obvious on the plain film
- The periosteum may be elevated by tumour invading through the cortex to produce a Codman's triangle

Further imaging
- US shows tumour bone formation with disordered vascularity
- Bone scan and chest CT for distant staging. Soft tissue deposits will also take up tracer
- MR is required for local staging. The possibility of skip lesions necessitates imaging the whole of a long bone
- Imaging-guided biopsy

Non-radiological investigations
- Histology
- Raised ESR and alkaline phosphatase

Management Generally consists of radical surgery combined with adjuvant chemotherapy (both often given preoperatively to shrink tumour prior to surgery). There is an approximately 50% 5-year survival rate, with no difference between amputation and limb-sparing surgery. Extremity tumours have a better prognosis and tibial lesions have a better survival rate than central lesions. Radiotherapy is used to control tumour at inoperable sites.

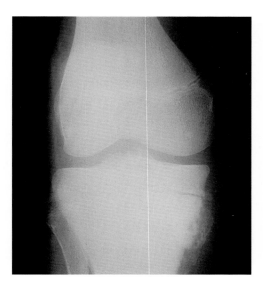
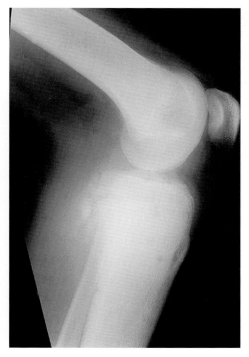

Fig 79.1 **AP and lateral knee.** There is tumour new bone formation extending into the soft tissues posteriorly at the proximal tibial metaphysis, destruction of the adjacent cortex and increased density in the metaphysis. There is an impression of soft tissue swelling that extends beyond the tumour bone formation.

80 Paget's disease (osteitis deformans)

Characteristics
- **Age range:** A disease of the elderly
- **Gender:** M:F = 2:1
- **Incidence:** 3% of individuals over the age of 40, 10% over 85 years
- **Pathology:** There is increased bone turnover with remodelling and expansion. Both osteoblastic and osteoclastic activity are increased. The bone is usually brittle as the internal architecture is abnormal. The cause is unknown, although the presence of inclusion bodies suggests a possible viral cause.

Clinical presentation It is commonly asymptomatic but may cause pain or noticeable deformity. It may be localized to part or the whole of one bone, most commonly the pelvis and tibia, followed by the femur, skull, spine and clavicle. The patient may present with complications of the disease which include nerve compression, particularly of the cranial nerves, spinal stenosis, fracture, high-output cardiac failure or hypercalcaemia. One percent of patients affected for 10 years or more develop a sarcoma, often heralded by increasing, uncontrollable pain.

Radiology
Description
- Affected bones show coarse trabeculation, increased density and enlargement
- The initial changes may be lytic
- Platybasia (Tam O'Shanter skull)
- Any bone in the body may be affected
- Microfractures may be seen, particularly when there is marked bowing

- Osteosarcoma formation may be evidenced by florid new bone formation with cortical destruction

Further imaging
- MR often shows a bizarre appearance with marked signal increase on T2 weighting and therefore is not always helpful in excluding malignancy
- CT may demonstrate the mixed tumour bone formation and destruction seen in malignancy and guide biopsy

Non-radiological investigations
- Raised plasma alkaline phosphatase
- Increased hydroxyproline excretion in the urine
- Hypercalcaemia, especially in immobilized patients

Management The majority of patients require no treatment. Associated arthritis often responds to non-steroidal antiinflammatories. Persistent bone pain, neurological complications, repeated fractures, high-output cardiac failure and hypercalcaemia require treatment with agents to suppress bone turnover, e.g. calcitonin and the diphosphonates. Disease activity can be monitored by alkaline phosphatase levels. Surgery is reserved for pathological fractures, painful osteoarthritis, nerve entrapment and spinal stenosis. Rarely, secondary osteosarcoma may be resectable, although the prognosis is extremely poor.

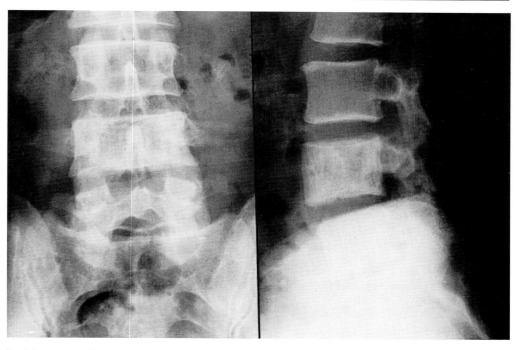

Fig 80.1 **AP and lateral lumbar spine.** There is a coarse trabecular pattern within an increase in density and expansion of the lumbar vertebrae.

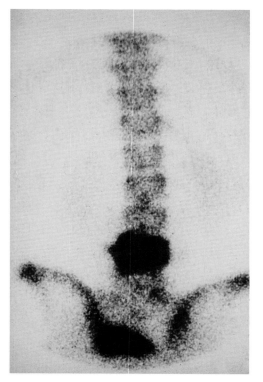

Fig 80.2 **Bone scan.** Note the markedly increased uptake in the fourth lumbar vertebra.

81 **Parosteal osteosarcoma**

Characteristics
- **Age range:** An older age group than osteosarcoma, generally middle aged
- **Gender:** Slight female preponderance
- **Incidence:** 4% of all osteosarcomas
- **Pathology:** Low-grade osteosarcoma. The tumour usually partially or completely encircles the shaft of the underlying bone. It metastasizes rarely and late.

Clinical presentation Classically it affects the distal posterior femur (72%). The proximal humerus and proximal tibia are the next most common sites. It presents as a slowly enlarging mass and is occasionally associated with pain. In contrast to osteosarcoma, the duration of symptoms varies from months to years.

Radiology
Description
- ☞ Dense, cloud-like new bone formation is seen, commonly at the distal femur
- The bone formation appears mature

- In aggressive lesions, rarely, cortical destruction can be identified

Further imaging
- Biopsy is generally guided by CT or fluoroscopy
- MR is required for local staging
- The lesions rarely metastasize but thoracic CT and bone scan may be indicated

Non-radiological investigations
- Histology

Management Wide excision is necessary and limb-sparing procedures are often performed due to its distal location, low grade and lack of local invasion. Rarely, amputation may be necessary. Systemic chemotherapy is recommended postoperatively for high-grade tumours. The 5-year survival rate is 75–85%.

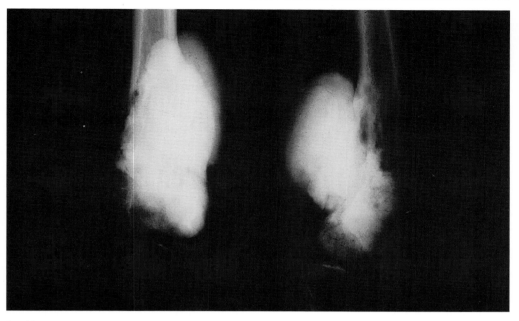

Fig 81.1 **AP and lateral knee.** There is dense mature new bone formation concentrically around the distal femur.

82 **Perthes disease**

Characteristics
- **Age range:** Peak incidence between 4 and 9 years
- **Gender:** M:F = 4:1
- **Incidence:** 1 in 10 000
- **Pathology:** Avascular necrosis of the femoral head. Unclear pathogenesis. Probably related to the transition of femoral head blood supply between the ages of 4 and 7 years.

Clinical presentation The child will have a constant or recurrent pain and limp. There is a decreased range of movement of the hip (especially abduction and internal rotation). ✳ Bilateral in 10%.

Radiology
Description
- Widening of joint space (may be earliest sign)
- 🔑 Small flattened femoral epiphysis
- Sclerosis of epiphysis
- Lucent areas in metaphysis
- Subcortical fracture (may only be seen on frog lateral view)
- Premature fusion of epiphysis
- Sclerotic fragmentation of femoral head
- Remodelling of femoral head

Further imaging
- Bone scan: decreased uptake in the early avascular phase and increased uptake later indicating repair or secondary degenerative change.
- MR: appearances depend on the phase. The femoral head may be of high signal on T2 early on, progressing to low signal intensity on T1 and T2 in the sclerotic repair phase. Fluid may be seen in a subchondral fracture.

Non-radiological investigations
- None

Management Initial bed rest until the pain subsides. If less than half of the head is involved radiologically then conservative treatment is indicated. Greater head involvement is an indication for 'containment', i.e. abduction plaster or splint, femoral or pelvic innominate osteotomy to contain the femoral head within the acetabulum. Best prognosis is when less than half the femoral head is involved and in female patients who are less than 6 years old.

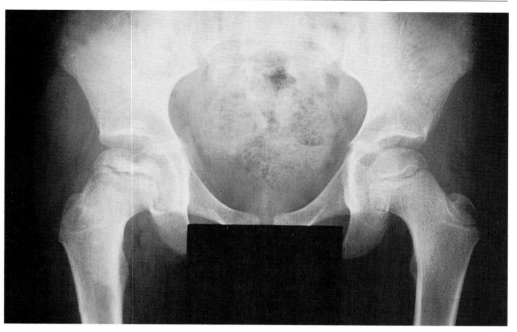

Fig 82.1 **AP pelvis.** Note the flattened and fragmented right femoral head with mixed sclerosis and lysis.

83 **Pigmented villonodular synovitis**

Characteristics
- **Age range:** Most common in the second to fourth decades, but present in wide age range
- **Gender:** More common in females
- **Incidence:** Rare
- **Pathology:** There is proliferation of the synovium with formation of villi and nodules. The tumour is golden brown in colour due to haemosiderin deposition. Microscopically there is hypertrophic synovium with fibroblasts, histiocytes and multinucleated giant cells.

Clinical presentation Patients present with pain, joint swelling, thickened synovium and an effusion. It most commonly affects the knee (75–90%) followed by the hip and ankle joint.

Radiology
Description
- Smooth bone erosion may be seen, often on both sides of a joint

Further imaging
- US shows a proliferative, frond-like pattern in the synovium
- ☞ MR also demonstrates proliferative synovial changes which are characteristically of low signal on both T1 and T2 weighting due to haemosiderin deposition
- Imaging-guided biopsy may rarely be appropriate

Non-radiological investigations
- Histology

Management Surgical excision is indicated – local excision for small lesions but synovectomy for extensive tumours. Incomplete synovectomy may be combined with radiotherapy. Although local recurrence is high, malignant change does not occur. Repeated recurrences and/or extensive bony destruction may necessitate arthroplasty or arthrodesis.

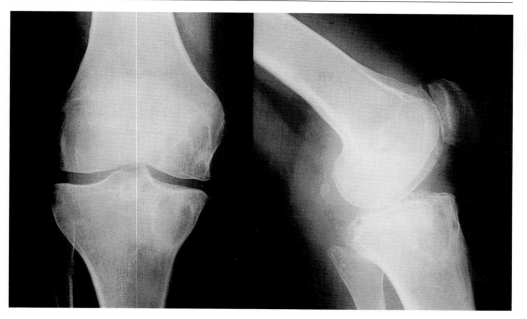

Fig 83.1 **AP and lateral knee.** There are well-defined large erosions on either side of the joint. An increase in soft tissue density is seen posterior to the joint.

84 **Plasmacytoma**

Characteristics

- **Age range:** Most common in the fourth and fifth decades, with a slightly younger profile than myeloma
- **Gender:** M = F
- **Incidence:** Less common than myeloma
- **Pathology:** A focal accumulation of marrow plasma cells, similar to myeloma but localized.

Clinical Presentation Most commonly seen in the spine, ribs, sternum, femora or humeri, presenting with a mass or pathological fracture. On occasion, may be exclusively soft tissue, usually in the head and neck. ✳ May disseminate and behave more aggressively, like myeloma.

Radiology

Description

- ☞ A markedly expansile, solitary, osteolytic lesion with trabeculations which give it a 'soap bubble' appearance
- May very rarely be sclerotic
- Intermediate zone of transition
- Frequently undergoes pathological fracture

Further imaging

- Imaging-guided biopsy

Non-radiological investigations

- Paraproteins should not be present in the plasma

Management Local radiotherapy combined with internal fixation if necessary. The surgical cavity can be packed with methylmethacrylate cement.

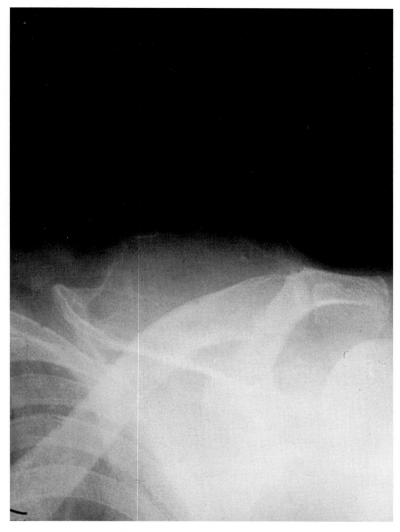

Fig 84.1 **AP shoulder.** There is an expansile 'soap bubble' lesion in the superior aspect of the scapula.

85 **Posterior cruciate ligament (PCL) tear**

Characteristics
- **Age range:** Young adults
- **Gender:** M >F
- **Incidence:** 3–20% of all ligament injuries. A common lesion although some are undetected; 2% of all American college football students are PCL deficient.
- **Pathology:** The PCL consists of large anterolateral and small posteromedial bands; it is intraarticular but extrasynovial. Can be torn by hyperextension or hyperflexion injuries of the knee (with or without varus/valgus force) or classic 'dashboard' injury (the dashboard forces the tibia posteriorly). The PCL does not heal.

Clinical presentation The history of injury is as above. Pain is generally felt posteriorly. A number of patients will present with instability. Clinical tests are for posterior sag, posterior draw or reverse pivot shift. Also, the patient should be assessed for posterolateral and posteromedial instability (posterior draw with foot externally and internally rotated 15° respectively).

Radiology
Description
- In an acute injury the plain film may show an effusion
- ☞ MR shows abnormal or absent signal in the PCL

Further imaging
- None

Non-radiological investigations
- None

Management The majority of isolated PCL injuries can be managed conservatively with rehabilitation physiotherapy. Bracing or orthoses can be useful. PCL reconstruction is generally recommended for young active patients with more than 10 mm of posterior tibial draw and symptomatic instability. Middle third of patellar tendon or hamstring grafts are used, though some surgeons prefer fresh-frozen Achilles tendon allograft. Acute injuries of the posterolateral corner should generally be surgically repaired within 3 weeks of the initial injury.

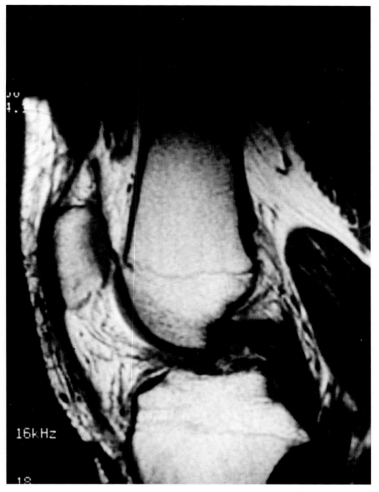

Fig 85.1 **T1-weighted sagittal MR of the knee.** The signal from the PCL is grossly abnormal.

86 **Psoriatic arthropathy**

Characteristics
- **Age range:** Any age, but the mean age of onset is 28 years
- **Gender:** M = F
- **Incidence:** Less than 5% of patients with psoriasis
- **Pathology:** A chronic papulosquamous, proliferative skin disease with a strong genetic component.

Clinical presentation The thoracolumbar junction, sacroiliac joints, hips, hands and feet are most commonly affected by the associated arthropathy. Skin lesions usually, but not invariably, precede the arthritis. These are red plaques, topped by silvery scales in hair-bearing areas, usually affecting the extensor surface of joints. Nail pitting is often present.

Radiology
Description
- Predilection for the distal interphalangeal joints
- Bone density is preserved
- ☞ Proliferative new bone formation is seen

- Erosions are present at joint surfaces
- There is a florid enthesopathy
- Ankylosis may be seen
- Asymmetrical sacroiliitis
- ☀ Severe destructive arthritis leading to 'cup and pencil' or 'main-en-lorgnette' deformities are seen

Further imaging
- None

Non-radiological investigations
- Rheumatoid negative
- HLA B27 positive in 50% (especially those with sacroiliitis)

Management Skin lesions are treated with topical preparations and in some cases steroids or immunosuppressives (azathioprine or methotrexate). Non-steroidal antiinflammatories and splintage to try to prevent deformity can alleviate joint symptoms. Immunosuppressives may rarely be used for joint disease. If severe, joint replacement or fusion may be performed.

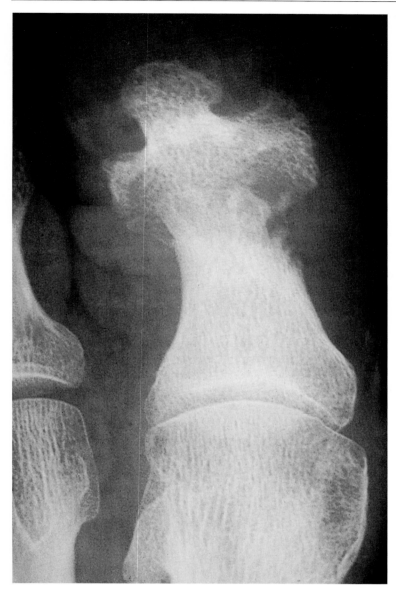

Fig 86.1 **DP great toes.** Erosive joint destruction is seen at the interphalangeal joint with fluffy new bone formation.

87 **Radiation necrosis**

Characteristics
- **Age range:** Any, following radiotherapy
- **Gender:** M = F
- **Incidence:** Uncommon
- **Pathology:** Prolonged or intense radiotherapy may cause bone death and the damage is dose related. It is due to the combined effect of damage to the microvascular, marrow and bone cells, all of which die. There may be no structural changes in bone for years. There is no repair or remodelling.

Clinical presentation Pain is the usual complaint and joints are stiff. Local signs, e.g. skin pigmentation and induration, may be present, as well as markers, 'tattoos', for the radiotherapy field. Common sites are shoulder and ribs (breast cancer), sacrum and hip and mandible. There is a high incidence of malignant change after at least 10 years, particularly osteosarcoma and MFH.

Radiology
Description
- Patchy loss of bone density with areas of sclerosis
- Non-anatomical, i.e. geometric, distribution
- Avascular necrosis with infarcts and subchondral lucency and collapse
- Extensive bone destruction may suggest malignant change

Further imaging
- MR and imaging-guided biopsy if malignancy is suspected

Non-radiological investigations
- Histology

Management Depends on the site of necrosis, quality of surrounding bone and life expectancy of the patient. If pain cannot be well controlled then joint replacement is justified, though results are inferior to prostheses in normal bone.

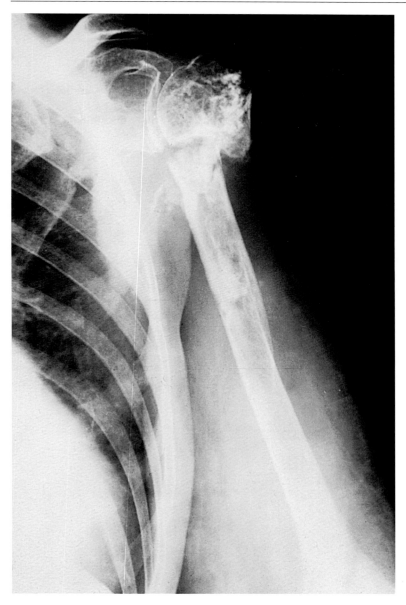

Fig 87.1 **AP shoulder.** There is a mixture of sclerosis and lysis in a geometric distribution corresponding to the radiation port. There has been a pathological fracture which has undergone non-union.

88 **Reiter's syndrome**

Characteristics
- **Age range:** Young adults
- **Gender:** 98% in males
- **Incidence:** Uncommon
- **Pathology:** The condition is of uncertain aetiology but presents following sexually transmitted disease or enteric infection; 76% of patients are HLA B27 positive.

Clinical presentation There is an asymmetrical arthritis associated with uveitis and urethritis. Cutaneous lesions (keratoderma blenorrhagica) and balanitis are characteristic. It is usually self-limiting, lasting 6 weeks to 6 months, but recurrences occur in up to 50%.

Radiology
Description
- Bone density is preserved

- Soft tissue swelling occurs around affected joints
- 🔑 Proliferative bone formation is present
- Feet are affected more often than the hands
- Unilateral sacroiliitis

Further imaging
- None

Non-radiological investigations
- HLA B27 positive
- 'Reiter cells' in joint aspirate
- ESR/CRP raised in the acute phase

Management Antibiotics are indicated in active urogenital or gut infection. Other treatment is supportive and symptomatic. Long-term NSAIDs may be necessary while waiting for remission.

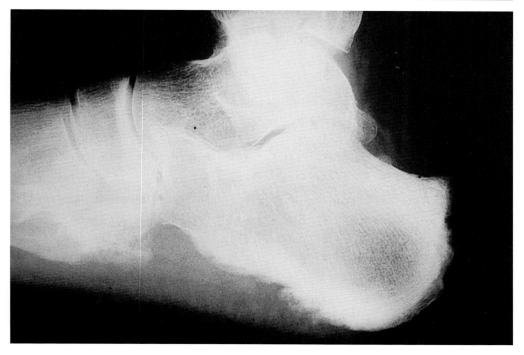

Fig 88.1 **Lateral ankle.** There is extensive periosteal new bone formation around the calcaneum and mid-foot.

89 **Renal bone disease**

Characteristics

- **Age range:** Depends on the aetiology of the underlying renal disease
- **Gender:** M = F
- **Incidence:** Now rare because of better management of chronic uraemia
- **Pathology:** Changes of secondary hyperparathyroidism are superimposed on those of osteomalacia. Renal insufficiency affects vitamin D metabolism, slowing intestinal calcium absorption while phosphate retention lowers calcium which increases parathormone production. Excessive maturation of osteoblasts leads to new bone formation and increasing amounts of osteoid are laid down, particularly in areas of high blood supply. Elevated calcium levels lead to calcification of this osteoid.

Clinical presentation There is a predisposition to fractures, particularly of the vertebrae and ribs, which may persist after transplantation. When renal osteodystrophy was more common, screening was carried out on patients with chronic renal failure by macroradiography of the hands.

Radiology

Description

- ☞ Increased bone density, particularly at the endplates, leads to a 'rugger jersey' spine
- Diffuse increase in bone density with ill-defined trabeculae
- Subperiosteal bone resorption
- Periostitis in long bones
- Ectopic calcification in vessels and soft tissues
- ☀ Avascular necrosis (AVN)

Further imaging

- MRI for AVN

Non-radiological investigations

- Low calcium and high serum phosphate

Management Transplantation may reverse the changes. Vitamin D and phosphate binders may alleviate the condition but parathyroidectomy may be necessary in tertiary hyperparathyroidism.

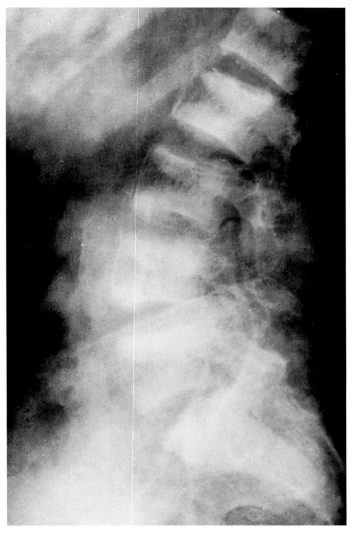

Fig 89.1 **Lateral lumbar spine.** Dense bands of sclerosis are seen – a 'rugger jersey' spine.

90 **Rheumatoid arthritis**

Characteristics
- **Age range:** Most commonly presents in the fifth and sixth decades
- **Gender:** Under 40 years M:F = 1:3, over 40 years M = F
- **Incidence:** Common, up to 3% of the population
- **Pathology:** The exact cause is unknown, although it is a chronic inflammatory disease and there is an abnormal immunological reaction. Anti-IgG antibodies and rheumatoid factor are present. The initial pathology is synovitis which, if left untreated, leads to joint and tendon destruction and subsequent deformity.

Clinical presentation Often insidious with non-specific symptoms such as tiredness, malaise, weight loss and intermittent muscle pain and weakness. Arthritis and synovitis are often symmetrical and classically affect MCP and proximal interphalangeal joints of the hands, wrists and MTP joints of the feet. Morning stiffness is common. Nodules on the extensor surfaces of the forearm and olecranon occur in 20% of cases and may also occur on tendon sheaths and in lungs or myocardium. Scleritis and pericardial or pleural effusions may occur and the patient may have a peripheral or entrapment neuropathy such as carpal tunnel syndrome.

Radiology
Description
- Soft tissue swelling may be seen on plain films
- Loss of bone density, starting in a periarticular distribution
- Symmetrical changes
- ☞ Erosions at joints and of the odontoid peg (requiring preoperative flexion and extension views)
- Subluxations, particularly at the MCP and MTP joints and in the cervical spine
- Concentric joint space loss
- Secondary degenerative change

Further imaging
- 🔔 MR to evaluate the soft tissues of the cervical spine and potential cord compression
- US for tendon ruptures and soft tissue masses
- Abdominal US in Felty's syndrome to measure the spleen
- CXR may show nodules, fibrosis, effusions and superior rib notching

Non-radiological investigations
- Full blood count shows anaemia of chronic disease
- ESR/CRP are raised
- Rheumatoid and antinuclear factors are positive in 70% and 30% of cases respectively, although neither is specific and may be negative in the early stages of disease
- Synovial biopsy may be helpful although the findings are usually non-specific

Management Inflamed joints should be rested or splinted in a functional position. Exercise and physiotherapy are important to maintain joint mobility and muscle strength. Occupational therapists can help by altering the patient's surroundings. NSAIDs are useful for pain but do not modify the course of the disease. Disease-modifying drugs include gold, penicillamine and hydroxychloroquine, steroids and methotrexate, all of which may have substantial side-effects. Local steroid injections into joints or tendon sheaths may be used. Surgery is used in the form of synovectomy for the wrist, fingers and elbow, tendon repair or transfer, excision arthroplasty (e.g. metatarsal heads), arthroplasty or fusion for the cervical spine. Ten percent of patients recover fully after the first attack of synovitis, 60% have recurrent attacks, 20% have severe joint disease requiring multiple operations, 10% are completely disabled.

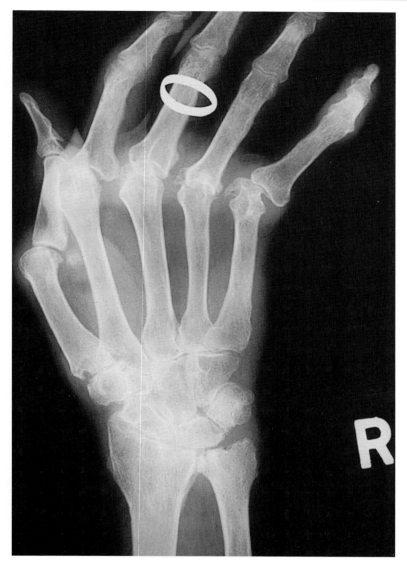

Fig 90.1 **DP hand.** There is a combination of reduction in bone density, erosions and multiple subluxations.

91 **Rickets**

Characteristics
- **Age range:** Most common age of presentation is between 4 and 18 months
- **Gender:** M = F
- **Incidence:** Not uncommon
- **Pathology:** Generally due to a deficiency of vitamin D or its metabolism, e.g. nutritional deficiency, lack of sunlight, malabsorption, liver disease (decreased 25-hydroxylation) and renal disease (decreased 1α-hydroxylation). Normal bone matrix fails to mineralize and histologically there is excess osteoid.

Clinical presentation
The child may present with delayed growth, bony deformity, enlarged epiphyses in long bones, proximal myopathy, enlarged costochondral junctions (rickety rosary), lateral indentation of the chest (Harrison's sulcus) and deformities of the skull – craniotabes. Bow legs are common, although knock knees or asymmetrical changes do occur. Hypocalcaemia may result in tetany, convulsions, carpopedal spasm and stridor.

Radiology
Description
- Most marked changes are seen at sites of bone growth and at weight-bearing areas

- Provisional zone of calcification becomes indistinct, resulting in an irregular, wide, 'frayed' metaphysis
- Epiphyses and apophyses may become indistinct
- Bowing of the legs and protrusio acetabuli may occur

Further imaging
- Increased metaphyseal uptake may be seen on bone scanning

Non-radiological investigations
- Plasma calcium is normal or low
- Plasma phosphate is low
- Alkaline phosphatase is high
- Urinary calcium excretion is very low
- In vitamin D deficiency plasma 25-hydroxylated vitamin D is low

Management
Treatment of the underlying cause is indicated. Generally large doses of calcium and vitamin D are given so the biochemistry needs careful monitoring during treatment. Hypophosphataemic rickets may require phosphate replacement.

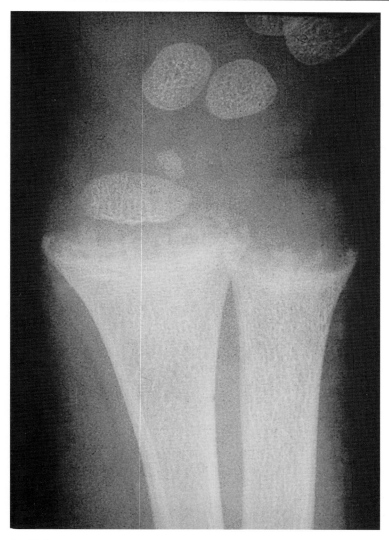

Fig 91.1 **AP wrist.** There is unmineralized osteoid at the growth plate with splaying and fraying of the metaphyses.

92 **Rotator cuff tear**

Characteristics
- **Age range:** Middle age and elderly
- **Gender:** M = F
- **Incidence:** Very common (60% of 60+-year-olds have small tears)
- **Pathology:** May be an acute injury or, more commonly, is secondary to subacromial impingement syndrome and chronic tendonitis of the cuff leading to degeneration. Supraspinatus is most often affected, although infraspinatus, teres minor and rarely subscapularis can be involved.

Clinical presentation An acute tear may present following an injury with sudden pain and weakness. A tear developing in chronic tendonitis may be asymptomatic or heralded by worsening pain and weakness. The pain is worst in the mid-arc of abduction (approximately 40–130°). The passive range of movement should be full unless a secondary frozen shoulder is present. If the patient is seen several weeks after the tear then there may be very little pain but obvious weakness. There may be wasting of the affected muscle and tenderness at the front of the shoulder.

Radiology
Description
- Plain films may be normal

- In chronic tears the humeral head may ride up into the subacromial space

Further imaging
- ☞ US is sensitive to partial as well as full-thickness tears as the supraspinatus tendon is well seen. The tear appears as a well-defined hypoechoic defect
- MR also demonstrates partial and full-thickness tears by alteration of signal in the rotator cuff and sometimes retraction of the supraspinatus muscle

Non-radiological investigations
- None

Management Asymptomatic tears require no treatment. The acute large tear should be repaired, especially in patients under 65. Acromioplasty should be performed at the same time to protect the repair. Large cuff tears may require mobilization of the cuff or even muscle transfer, e.g. latissimus dorsi. In the patient (predominantly elderly) whose main problem is pain rather than weakness, physiotherapy and subacromial steroid injections are useful, similar to the treatment of tendonitis without tear. Resistant pain in these cases may benefit from acromioplasty which may be done arthroscopically and debridement of the cuff without repair.

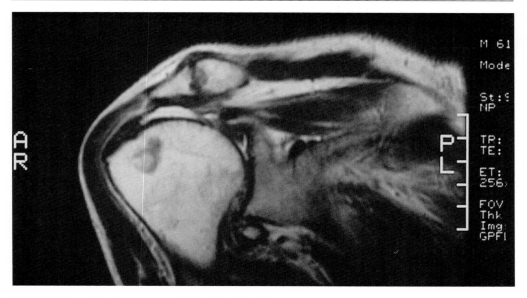

Fig 92.1 **T2-weighted paracoronal MR of the shoulder.** There is degenerative change in the acromioclavicular joint and a small bright effusion in the subacromial space. There is a 'bare area' where the supraspinatus tendon should be. Note also the degenerative cyst in the humeral head.

93 **Sarcoidosis**

Characteristics

- **Age range:** Presents in the third to fifth decades
- **Gender:** M:F = 1:3
- **Incidence:** Six cases per 100 000 population, 14 times more common in patients of black origin
- **Pathology:** A multisystem disease of unknown aetiology. Histology shows non-caseating granulomas.

Clinical presentation
The acute form presents with bilateral hilar lymphadenopathy, fever, rash and arthralgia. The chronic form presents with malaise, weakness and cough. Bone is involved in up to 20% of cases. ⚠ Twenty percent go on to irreversible pulmonary fibrosis.

Radiology
Description
- Marked soft tissue swelling produces a 'sausage digit'
- ⚷ Affected bone shows a 'lace-like' trabecular pattern
- Small lytic or cystic lesions are seen in the phalanges
- Destructive changes may develop

Further imaging
- CXR, chest CT, gallium scan and brain MRI may be necessary to assess overall disease activity

Non-radiological investigations
- Raised serum angiotensin-converting enzyme (sACE)
- Lung function
- Rarely, a Kveim test may be required

Management
Symptomatic, as most cases resolve spontaneously. Steroids may be given to reduce disease activity.

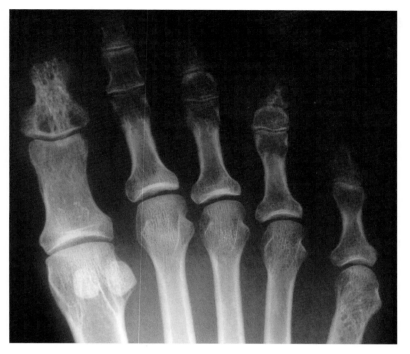

Fig 93.1 **DP toes.** There is a lytic process affecting several phalanges and the head of the little toe MT.

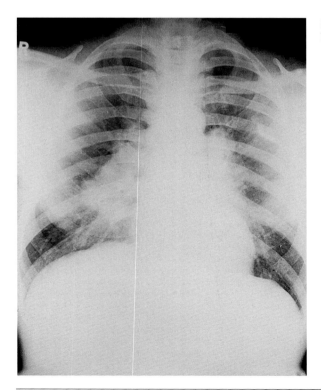

Fig 93.2 **PA chest.** There is massive bilateral hilar lymphadenopathy.

94 **Scheuermann's disease**

Characteristics

- **Age range:** Patients normally present at puberty
- **Gender:** M:F = 3:2
- **Incidence:** A frequent cause of back pain in adolescents
- **Pathology:** Often described as an osteochondritis although the cause is controversial. Other possible causes include avascular necrosis of the ring apophyses, traumatic infarction of the epiphyseal plates during the growth spurt and genetic transmission. It is characterized by vertebral wedging and subsequent growth disturbance of the endplate.

Clinical presentation The child often becomes increasingly 'round shouldered' and may complain of backache. Pain is most severe during the growth spurt. A smooth thoracic kyphosis is seen which is not correctable (distinguishing it from postural kyphosis). There is often an associated compensatory lordosis. Neurological examination is generally normal, though paraparesis can occur due to thoracic disc herniations or compression fractures. Cardiopulmonary dysfunction can occur with severe thoracic deformities.

Radiology

Description

- Wedge-shaped vertebral bodies
- Narrowed intervertebral discs which may calcify
- ☞ Poorly formed, irregular endplates with multiple nucleus pulposus herniations (Schmorl's nodes)
- Premature marginal osteophyte formation
- Progressive kyphosis

Further imaging

- None

Non-radiological investigations

- None

Management Usually conservative. Curves of 40–60° (without evidence of progression) require strengthening exercises and postural training. Bracing may be of benefit in curves of 50–75° in the skeletally immature patients. Surgery (anterior release, fusion and posterior instrumentation) may be considered in skeletally mature patients with a kyphosis of greater than 75° if they are experiencing pain, have an unacceptable cosmetic deformity or impending spastic paresis. Surgery has a high complication rate and spinal cord monitoring is essential. Postoperatively a brace is required for 6 months or until anterior fusion is confirmed on radiographs.

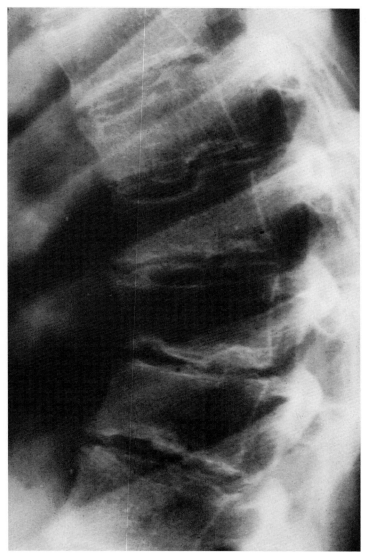

Fig 94.1 **Lateral thoracic spine.** There is a kyphosis associated with generalized endplate irregularity.

95 **Scleroderma**

Characteristics
- **Age range:** Most often presents in the fourth to sixth decades
- **Gender:** M:F = 1:3
- **Incidence:** Rare
- **Pathology:** An autoimmune disease where there is progressive fibrosis and tightening of the skin for which the cause is unknown.

Clinical presentation Skin disease may be the only abnormality, although it may be part of CREST syndrome (Calcinosis of subcutaneous tissues, Raynaud's phenomenon, decreased oesophageal motility, Sclerodactyly and Telangiectasia). There may be polyarthritis and myopathy.
☀ Generalized progressive systemic sclerosis may affect the kidney, leading to severe hypertension, the lung, leading to fibrosis, and the gastrointestinal tract.

Radiology
Description
- 🔑 Soft tissue atrophy in the hand is associated with calcification in the pulp

- Acroosteolysis
- Soft tissue calcification is also seen around major joints

Further imaging
- Barium studies for associated gut abnormalities
- CXR/chest CT for lung fibrosis

Non-radiological investigations
- Antinuclear antibody (ANA) stains positive in a nucleolar pattern (CREST shows anticentromere ANA)
- ESR/CRP may be raised
- Anaemia of chronic disease is frequently seen

Management Steroids may be of benefit although often there is no effective treatment. Symptomatic support is needed and Raynaud's and pulp ulceration may be alleviated by sympathectomy.

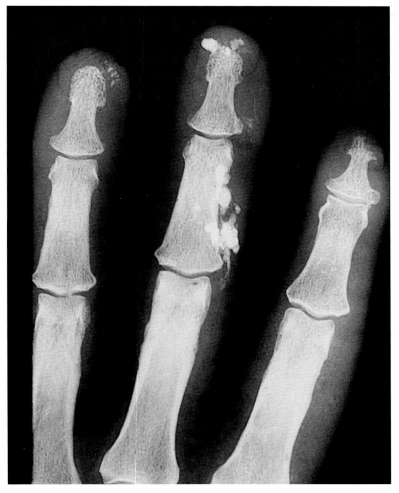

Fig 95.1 **DP phalanges.** There is soft tissue calcification with atrophic change affecting the ring finger terminal phalanx, and acroosteolysis.

96 **Scurvy**

Characteristics
- **Age range:** May occur at any age but now not seen outside childhood
- **Gender:** M = F
- **Incidence:** Extremely rare
- **Pathology:** Vitamin C (ascorbic acid) deficiency

Clinical presentation Children present with irritability and pain and may refuse to walk. There is gum swelling and haemorrhage into the skin. Damage to follicles leads to 'question mark' hairs.
🔔 The main differential diagnosis is NAI.

Radiology
Description
- ☞ Metaphyseal lucency associated with generalized demineralization
- Cortex remains dense and appears 'pencilled'
- Epiphyses show 'Wimberger's ring sign'
- Lateral metaphyseal 'Pelkan's' spurs occur at the distal femur due to metaphyseal fractures
- Periosteal reactions due to extensive subperiosteal haemorrhage

Further imaging
- None

Non-radiological investigations
- Full blood count for anaemia
- Calcium, phosphate and alkaline phosphatase are normal
- Clotting is normal

Management Vitamin C is given together with blood transfusions. Leukaemia, syphilis and metastatic neuroblastoma must also be excluded as differential diagnoses.

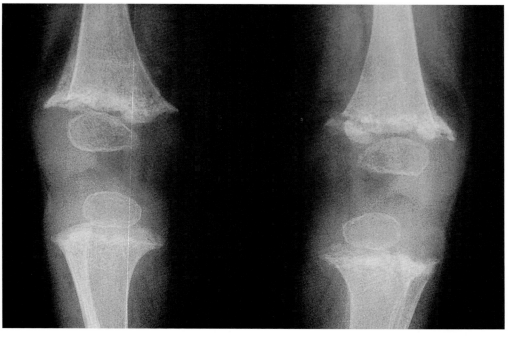

Fig 96.1 **AP knees.** There is reduction in the bone density with sharp preservation of the cortical outline of the distal femoral epiphyses. Pelkan's spurs are also seen.

97 **Septic arthritis**

Characteristics
- **Age range:** Any age
- **Gender:** M = F
- **Incidence:** Uncommon
- **Pathology:** Occurs secondary to direct invasion (penetrating wound, injection or surgery), by extension of osteomyelitis or bone abscess or by haematogenous spread. The causal organism is usually *Staph. aureus,* though *Haemophilus influenzae* is common in infants and *Neisseria gonorrhoeae* in young, sexually active adults.

Clinical presentation Typical presentation is with monoarthritis, most commonly in the knee followed by the hip, fever, swelling and limitation of movement. Infants often present with septicaemia.

Radiology
Description
- Effusion may be evident on the plain radiograph, depending on the joint involved
- Periarticular osteoporosis
- Cortical destruction after 10–14 days
- Healing may occur with fusion
- ⚜ Epiphyseal damage in children may result in a classic 'chevron' deformity

Further imaging
- ⚷ US/MRI shows effusions and US allows aspiration
- Isotope scans may show early changes, unless high joint pressure prevents isotope reaching the epiphysis in children
- MRI may demonstrate oedema in adjacent bone

Non-radiological investigations
- Aspirate sent for MC+S
- ESR/CRP raised
- White cell count raised
- Blood cultures are positive in approximately 70% of cases

Management Aspiration of the joint, Gram stain and culture are essential. Treatment consists of parenteral antibiotics (flucloxacillin in adults with the addition of cephalosporins in children) which are changed according to sensitivities. The joint should be washed out, arthroscopically if appropriate or by an open procedure, and the affected joint should be rested in a splint. Long-term sequelae include secondary osteoarthritis and extensive joint destruction and permanent deformity.

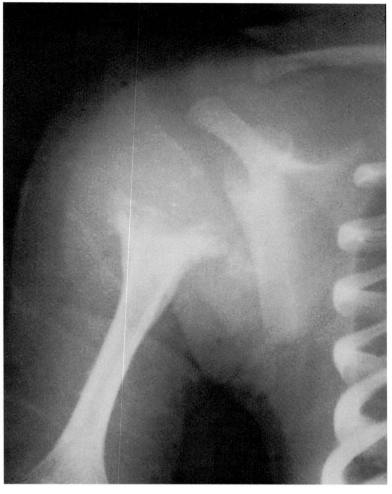

Fig 97.1 **AP shoulder.** The epiphysis has been destroyed. There is chronic change at the metaphysis with sclerosis and modelling abnormality. The beginning of a 'chevron' deformity is seen.

98 Shoulder instability

Characteristics
- **Age range:** All age groups
- **Gender:** M:F = 9:1 in the younger age group, M:F = 1:3 in older patients
- **Incidence:** Common, 1.7% of individuals
- **Pathology:** May be anterior (>95%), posterior (3.8%), multidirectional or inferior. It may also be voluntary or habitual. Stability is achieved in the normal joint through osseous and cartilaginous joint surfaces, lateral and ligamentous structures and surrounding muscles. Failure of or injury to these structures can result in instability. Ligamentous laxity may also be associated with instability.

Clinical presentation
The patient frequently presents with an acute traumatic dislocation with a history of injury and a deformed shoulder. Posterior dislocations may be readily missed and a key sign is loss of external rotation or fixed internal rotation. Chronic instability is difficult to diagnose (especially posterior) and the patient may have apprehension. Young patients may present with a secondary subacromial impingement syndrome.

Radiology
Description
- Stryker's views may show a Hill-Sachs (or Hatchet) defect in the posterior part of the humeral head
- CT arthrography shows the degree of soft tissue as well as bony damage
- ☞ A Bankart lesion of the anterior glenoid labrum and anterior soft tissue stripping from the glenoid neck may be demonstrated

Further imaging
- The role of MR in evaluation of the unstable shoulder remains undefined; its value may be increased by either direct (intraarticular) or indirect (intravenous) gadolinium

Non-radiological investigations
- Arthroscopy is a useful diagnostic tool for observing the ligaments, labrum and articular surface to assess whether true mechanical instability is present.

Management
Acute dislocations require immediate reduction under general anaesthetic or sedation. Patients with subluxation and mild instability and voluntary dislocators are treated with physiotherapy and a strengthening exercise programme. Biofeedback is useful. Operative treatment is indicated for patients with recurrent non-voluntary dislocations, often with minimal trauma. The stabilization procedure performed is addressed to the direction of the instability and a combined anterior/posterior approach is occasionally required. Arthroscopic stabilization is sometime possible although results are inferior to open procedures with up to a 20% lower success rate. Postoperatively the shoulder is protected in a sling for 4–6 weeks and this is followed by a rehabilitation programme to regain strength, range of movement and coordination of the glenohumeral and scapulohumeral joints.

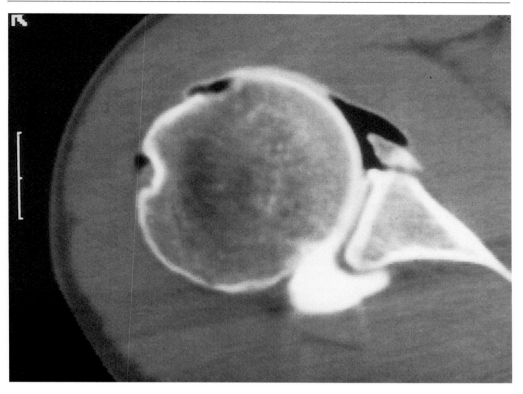

Fig 98.1 **CT arthrogram of the shoulder.** There is a fracture of the anterior glenoid and labrum but little anterior soft tissue disruption.

99 **Sickle cell disease**

Characteristics
- **Age range:** May present from infancy to adulthood
- **Gender:** M = F
- **Incidence:** Common in patients of black African origin
- **Pathology:** ☞ There is a severe haemolytic anaemia due to an amino acid substitution in the haemoglobin molecule (β6 Glu to Val).

Clinical presentation
Homozygous patients (ss) have sickle cell anaemia and are prone to acute crises from infection (commonly salmonella osteomyelitis), infarction or rarely haemolysis. It causes severe pain, often in bones, and may mimic an acute abdomen or pneumonia. Patients may present in infancy with jaundice or swollen hands and feet. ⚠ In later life, patients suffer renal failure, AVN and splenic infarction. Heterozygous patients (As) have no disability until subjected to hypoxia, e.g. general anaesthesia.

Radiology
Description
- Loss of bone density with a coarse trabecular pattern due to the increased medullary space
- Generalized increase in bone density may also occur
- Marrow hyperplasia leads to widening of the diploë
- Biconcave, 'H'-shaped vertebrae due to endplate AVN
- Bone destruction or sclerosis due to infection or, in older patient, infarction
- Premature growth plate closure may lead to deformities
- ☞ AVN of the humeral and femoral heads

Further imaging
- CXR may show mediastinal abnormalities due to extramedullary haemopoiesis and changes of heart failure
- Bone scan and MR may be necessary for the further evaluation of infection or infarction

Non-radiological investigations
- A full blood count shows anaemia – typically Hb 6–8 g/dl, reticulocytes 10–20%
- Serum electrophoresis – distinguishes ss from As forms

Management
Acute crises are treated with analgesia, fluids, O_2, antibiotics, blood or exchange transfusion. Pneumococcal vaccine is given and long-term low-dose penicillin V. Surgery may be necessary for sequestra and subperiosteal abscess in the case of bone infection. Joint replacement may be necessary for avascular necrosis.

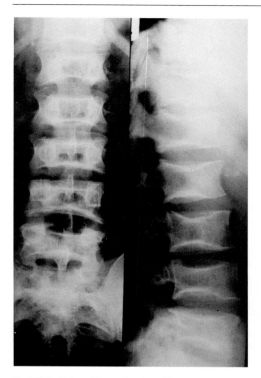

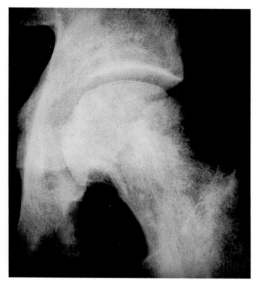

Fig 99.1 **AP and lateral spine.** There is symmetrical 'H'-shaped endplate depression of all the vertebral bodies.

Fig 99.2 **AP hip.** Avascular necrosis of the femoral head with a line of subchondral lucency on a background of patchy sclerosis. There is also flattening of the femoral heads.

100 Simple bone cyst

Characteristics
- **Age range:** 80% are seen in patients aged 3–19 years
- **Gender:** M:F = 3:1
- **Incidence:** Common
- **Pathology:** It is thought not to be a true neoplasm. The lining tissue varies from a thin fibrocartilaginous membrane to cellular tissue containing giant cells, chronic inflammatory cells and haemosiderin-laden macrophages.

Clinical presentation Usually discovered after it has undergone a pathological fracture or as an incidental finding on a radiograph. The most common sites are the proximal humerus (67%) and the proximal femur (15%).

Radiology
Description
- A well-defined, slightly expansile, lytic, metaphyseal lesion
- In older patients the lesion may 'migrate' to the mid-shaft
- Pathological fracture is very common and may lead to the 'falling fragment' sign

Further imaging
- CT and MR may rarely show fluid–fluid levels
- Imaging-guided biopsy

Non-radiological investigations
- Histology, although often only serous fluid is obtained from the lesion

Management Traditional treatment is by curettage, though local recurrence is common. In general it should be treated by aspiration, high-pressure meglumine diatrizoate injection and intracavity methylprednisolone. Recurrence can be treated with repeat injections. Pathological fractures should be allowed to heal before injection is performed. Less than 1% of simple bone cysts regress spontaneously.

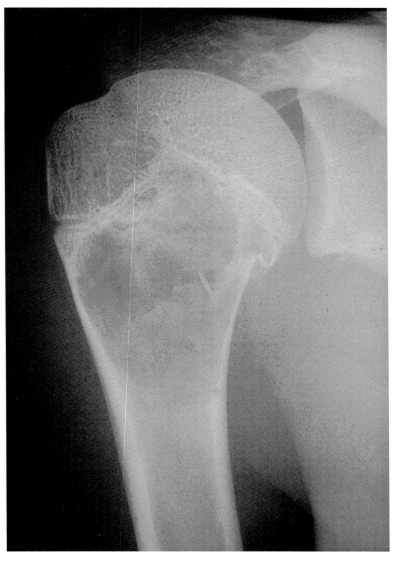

Fig 100.1 **AP shoulder.** A relatively well-defined lucent area is seen in the metaphysis. There is a pathological fracture and a small density within the lucency, the 'falling fragment' sign.

101 Slipped upper femoral epiphysis (SUFE)

Characteristics
- **Age range:** M 14–16 years, F 11–14 years
- **Gender:** M:F = 3:1
- **Incidence:** 2–3 cases per 100 000 per year
- **Pathology:** Possibly related to hormonal imbalance. The pituitary hormonal growth spurt may not be matched by gonadal hormone activity promoting physical maturation. Thirty percent of patients are obese and hypogonadal. It is rare in southern Asians and black Africans but more common in black Americans.

Clinical presentation Usually presents with limping and spontaneous pain in the groin, anterior thigh or knee; 50% of patients give a history of injury, 50% describe a gradual onset. On examination, the leg is externally rotated and short; 20% are bilateral.

Radiology
Description
- The epiphyseal plate is widened with metaphyseal irregularity
- 🔑 The epiphysis is usually displaced medially and posteriorly
- 🔆 Displacement may only be seen on the frog-leg view and this is therefore necessary if SUFE is suspected but not seen on the frontal view
- The angle between the neck and shaft of the femur is reduced
- Be aware of the complications of avascular necrosis and chondrolysis

Further imaging
- Ultrasound shows minimal displacement and an effusion
- Check the contralateral side

Non-radiological investigations
- None

Management Preserve blood supply, stabilize the physis and correct any deformity. For less than one-third slip, pin in situ; one-third to two-thirds slip, pin in situ possibly followed by osteotomy. For greater than two-thirds slip, open reduction, Dunn osteotomy or pin in situ and intertrochanteric triplane osteotomy.

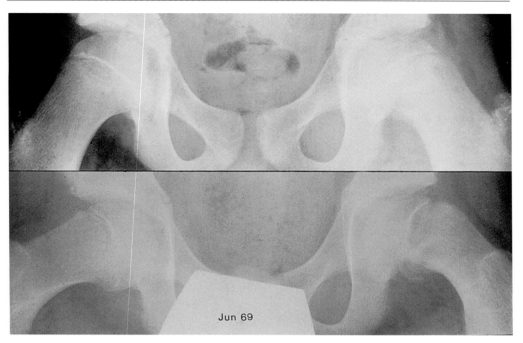

Jun 69

Fig 101.1 **AP and frog-leg lateral pelvis.** The changes on the AP view are subtle although a little widening of the growth plate is shown. The frog-leg lateral clearly shows the posteromedial slippage of the left epiphysis. There is also some metaphyseal lucency which is frequently seen in this condition.

102 **Spina bifida**

Characteristics

- **Age range:** Presents from birth and may be diagnosed antenatally
- **Gender:** M = F
- **Incidence:** 0.5% of all UK births (10× increase if an affected sibling, 30× increase if an affected parent)
- **Pathology:** There is failure of fusion of the posterior neural arch, most commonly in the lumbar spine. The contents of the vertebral canal may prolapse through the defect. A CSF-filled meningeal sac is termed a meningocoele, a sac containing neural tissue is called a myelomeningocoele. Spina bifida may be associated with diastematomyelia (split cord) (see p. 56) or lower limb deformities. Spina bifida occulta, where there is incomplete fusion of the posterior elements, is a common (5%) incidental finding of no clinical significance.

Clinical presentation Skin-covered defects may present at any age with cauda equina syndrome or urinary problems such as enuresis, incontinence or frequency. If a CSF sac is present it is obvious from birth. Hydrocephalus and a Chiari II malformation (herniation of the cerebellar tonsils) may be present in cases with myelomeningocoele, though may not appear until surgical closure of the defect. Closed defects do not have a significant incidence of associated cerebral anomalies. Neurological deficit is very variable and depends on the level and severity of the defect; paresis leads to gracile, osteopenic bones and pathological fractures are common. Lower limb deformities are common: hip dislocation, talipes and genu recurvatum. ⚠ Urinary tract problems develop in 90% of cases.

Radiology

Description

- Incomplete fusion of the posterior arch of the vertebrae is seen on plain films
- 🔑 Majority are diagnosed antenatally at the anomaly scan
- Meningocoele may be evident on a plain film

Further imaging

- US at birth to determine level of the cord and assess soft tissues
- MRI of the spine for full assessment of soft tissue and bone anomalies
- Head MRI to exclude associated cerebral abnormalities
- Renal tract US in later years to evaluate for hydronephrosis

Non-radiological investigations

- During pregnancy the open lesions result in raised α-foetoprotein levels in both the amniotic fluid and the blood

Management The incidence of spina bifida can be reduced by taking folic acid for the first 12 weeks' gestation. An antenatal diagnosis may result in a decision to terminate. Selection of patients for surgical closure is controversial so a team approach with surgeons and therapists is essential. Skin closure within 48 hours is the priority in patients with good prognostic signs and is followed by management of the hydrocephalus, then the associated deformities. Only one-third of patients achieve independent walking.

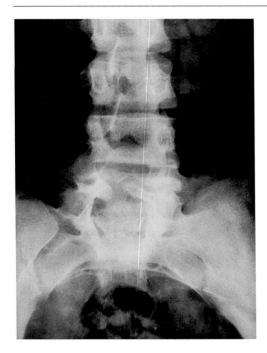

Fig 102.1 **AP lumbar spine.** There is failure of fusion of the posterior elements at L5 with a bizarre eccentric appearance to those above.

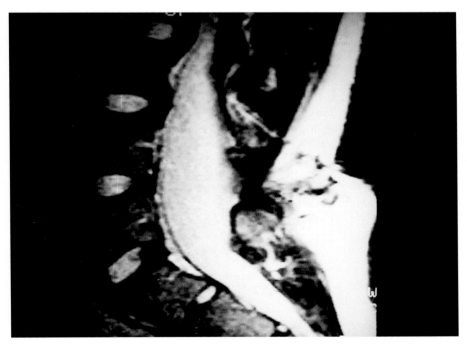

Fig 102.2 **T2-weighted sagittal spinal MRI.** The spinal canal is dilated in its distal part and a defect in the posterior elements can be seen. This is a covered defect, although some stranding is seen in the skin over the defect.

103 **Spondyloepiphyseal dysplasia (SED)**

Characteristics
- **Age range:** Bimodal; either presents in infancy or after 5 years of age
- **Gender:** M = F
- **Incidence:** Uncommon
- **Pathology:** Probably due to spontaneous mutations of the type II collagen gene. The congenita form is autosomal dominant, the tarda is X-linked recessive.

Clinical presentation The limbs and trunk are short with an increased thoracic kyphosis and lumbar lordosis.

Radiology
Description
- There is delayed appearance and maturity of ossification centres
- Dysplastic epiphyses and metaphyses
- Platyspondyly

- Kyphoscoliosis (especially in the tarda form)
- Hypoplastic odontoid peg
- Low, square ilium with a deep acetabulum
- Undertubulation of long bones
- Coxa vara and genu valgum

Further imaging
- None

Non-radiological investigations
- There is increased excretion of keratan sulphate in the urine

Management SED congenita may require corrective osteotomies for coxa vara or knee deformities and atlantoaxial fusion if there is odontoid hypoplasia. SED tarda patients need symptomatic relief for backache. Both may require custom-built total hip arthroplasties, due to the coxa vara.

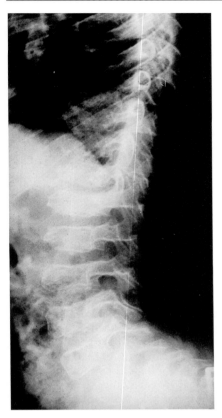

Fig 103.1 **Lateral spine.** Platyspondyly.

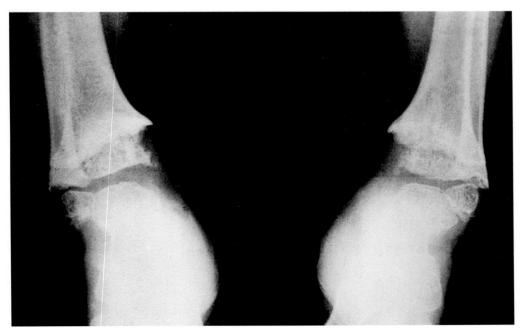

Fig 103.2 **AP ankles.** There is irregularity and mottling of the distal tibial epiphyses. Changes are also seen in the fibular epiphyses.

104 Spondylolysis (pars interarticularis defect)

Characteristics
- **Age range:** Most symptomatic patients are in the second and third decades
- **Gender:** M:F = 3:1
- **Incidence:** 3–7% of the population
- **Pathology:** There is a defect in the pars interarticularis, the gap being filled with fibrous tissue. May be congenital, when a familial association is sometimes seen, or due to a stress fracture. It is the commonest cause of spondylolisthesis.

Clinical presentation Back pain during exercise, although it may be an incidental finding. Radicular symptoms may occur. Lumbar movements are generally normal although there may be hamstring tightness.

Radiology
Description
- ☛ Lateral views of the lumbar spine show a defect of the pars interarticularis (broken neck of 'scottie dog'). The ability to identify this can sometimes be enhanced by oblique views
- This may or may not be associated with a slip (spondylolisthesis)
- Slips are classified into four grades: grade I up to 30% movement on the vertebral body below, grade II 30–60%, grade III 60–100% and grade IV when the superior vertebral body has slipped forward off the vertebral body below.

Further imaging
- When there is a high index of suspicion – straight or reverse gantry angle CT is the best method for demonstrating a defect or sclerosis with a healing defect
- Bone scanning shows a hot spot in healing or 'active' defect
- MR does not provide reliable information on spondylolysis

Non-radiological investigations
- None

Management Most patients can be managed conservatively with activity limitation, abdominal strengthening, hamstring stretching and antiinflammatory medication. Injury may result in an acute fracture of the pars and these patients may benefit from a plaster jacket for 3 months to allow the fracture to heal. Surgery is reserved for patients with disabling symptoms, greater than 50% or progressive slip and significant neurological compression. Posterior intertransverse fusion is recommended in children, although in adults posterior or anterior fusion is required (with or without reduction of the slip).

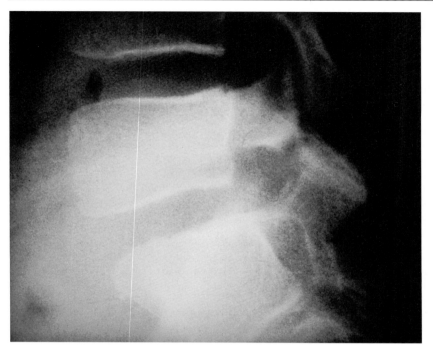

Fig 104.1 **Lateral lumbar spine.** A clear defect is seen in the pars interarticulares. There is minimal forward slip.

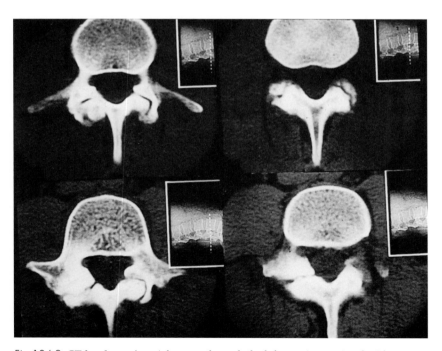

Fig 104.2 **CT lumbar spine.** A lucency through the left pars is associated with substantial sclerosis.

105 Subchondral cyst (geode)

Characteristics
- **Age range:** Middle age or elderly but may be seen in younger patients
- **Gender:** M = F
- **Incidence:** Very common
- **Pathology:** May be secondary to osteoarthritis, trauma or inflammatory arthritis, particularly rheumatoid. Cysts associated with crystal deposition disease may be very large. A breach in the articular cartilage allows intravasation of synovial fluid.

Clinical presentation Is that of the underlying condition. In particular, crystal pyrophosphate deposition disease presents with acute inflammatory episodes with effusions and pain.

Radiology
Description
- 🔑 Well-defined lytic lesion which reaches the articular surface
- Variable in size
- Joint space may be normal or reduced
- The roof of the cyst may 'collapse'
- In pyrophosphate deposition disease there may be chondrocalcinosis and an obvious effusion

Further imaging
- MRI shows the lesion to be filled with fluid

Non-radiological investigations
- Appropriate to the underlying cause
- Pyrophosphate crystals in joint fluid show negative birefringence

Management None is indicated for the cyst alone but associated degenerative or inflammatory arthritis may require treatment.

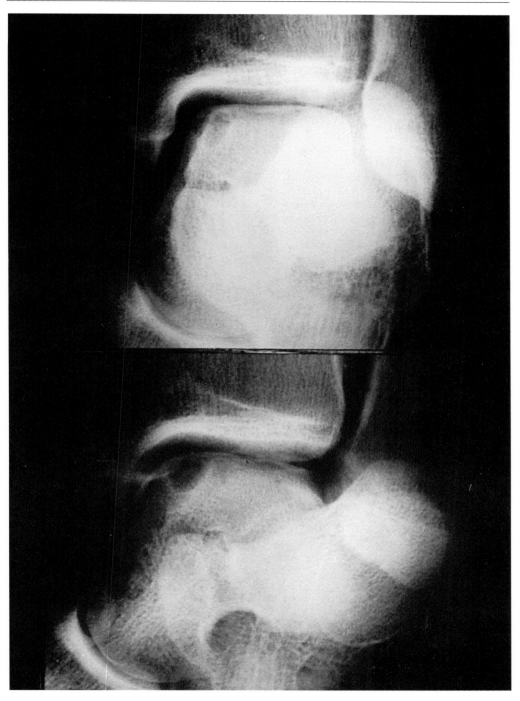

Fig 105.1 **AP and lateral ankle.** This is a posttraumatic subchondral cyst in the talar dome. Note the lucency with a sclerotic rim that sits just under the articular surface.

106 **Synovial chondromatosis**

Characteristics
- **Age range:** Most commonly seen in the fourth decade but may present at almost any age
- **Gender:** M:F = 2–4:1
- **Incidence:** Uncommon
- **Pathology:** Metaplasia of the synovium results in cartilaginous or osteocartilaginous nodules which may become loose within the joint. These may form conglomerates or reattach to the synovium. They may either continue to grow or reabsorb.

Clinical presentation Progressive, intermittent pain and limitation of movement. There is usually an effusion and there may be symptoms of a loose body such as locking. 70% of cases affect the knee, often in the presence of a Baker's cyst, and it is generally monoarticular. Rarely, it may occur in a tendon sheath or bursa.

Secondary degenerative change may be seen and malignant change has been reported ⚠ .

Radiology
Description
- ⚷ More than four loose bodies are defined as synovial chondromatosis
- These may remain attached to synovium or be completely loose
- Irregular, chondroid calcification can be seen around a joint

Further imaging
- MR and US may define the lesions more clearly

Non-radiological investigations
- None

Management Removal of the loose bodies and synovectomy to prevent recurrence.

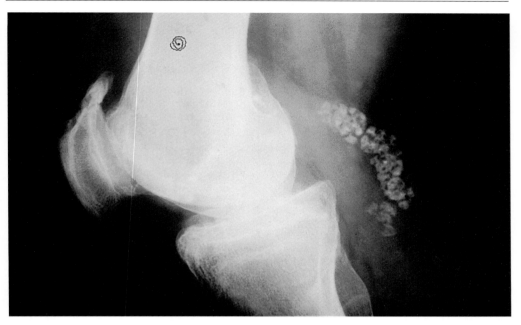

Fig 106.1 **Lateral knee.** There are multiple, faceted calcifications lying in a Baker's cyst posterior to the knee joint.

107 **Synovial sarcoma**

Characteristics
- **Age range:** Most common in the third to fifth decades
- **Gender:** M:F = 2:3
- **Incidence:** 10% of all soft tissue sarcomas
- **Pathology:** Classically has a biphasic population of spindle cells and epithelioid cells. Virtually all synovial sarcomas are high grade.

Clinical presentation Typically presents as a deep-seated, well-circumscribed, firm multinodular mass, seen around the knee. ⚠ Ninety percent are extraarticular and are seldom even contiguous with a synovial space.

Radiology
Description
- ☞ A well-defined soft tissue mass may be seen

- 30% show amorphous calcification on the plain film
- Adjacent bone may be porotic or demonstrate evidence of invasion, either remodelling or destruction

Further imaging
- Imaging-guided biopsy
- MRI for local staging
- Chest CT and bone scan for distant staging

Non-radiological investigations
- Histology

Management Small lesions can be treated by wide excision. However, most will need radical resection or amputation, together with radiotherapy and chemotherapy.

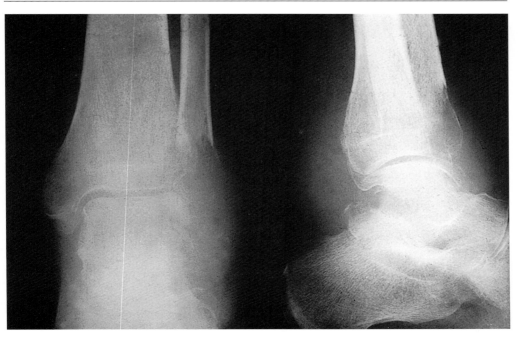

Fig 107.1 **AP and lateral ankle.** There is aggressive bony destruction affecting the fibula and adjacent bones. There is an associated soft tissue lesion.

108 Systemic lupus erythematosus (SLE)

Characteristics
- **Age range:** Most frequently seen in women of child-bearing age
- **Gender:** M:F = 1:10
- **Incidence:** 1 in 2000, three times more common in patients of black origin
- **Pathology:** A non-organ specific, autoimmune disease characterized by antinuclear antibodies and vasculitis. It may be triggered by viral infection in genetically predisposed individuals.

Clinical presentation It can affect any organ system and therefore the presentation is varied. Patients commonly present with musculoskeletal problems (arthralgia, myalgia and myositis), followed by cutaneous disease (butterfly rash on the face, alopecia, Raynaud's phenomenon and buccal ulceration). There may also be pyrexia of unknown origin, splenomegaly, renal, pulmonary or cardiac failure. Neurological symptoms are common due to the small vessel vasculitis.

Radiology
Description
- ⚷ Bone changes are minimal
- Loss of bone density with subchondral lucency
- Jaccoud's variant produces pseudosubluxation at the MCP joints

Further imaging
- CXR demonstrates small-volume lungs without fibrotic change although there may be small effusions
- Diffuse high-signal lesions are seen on brain MR in cerebrovascular disease

Non-radiological investigations
- 75% have a normochromic, normocytic leukaemia with lowered platelets and white cells
- Raised ESR/CRP
- Positive antinuclear antibody in 80%
- ⚷ Positive anti-double-stranded DNA is almost exclusive to SLE
- 40% positive rheumatoid factor
- 10% false-positive syphilis serology

Management Non-steroidal antiinflammatories may control early minor symptoms. Sun block reduces cutaneous disease. Uncontrolled symptoms may respond to hydroxychloroquine and steroids. Low dose steroids are appropriate maintenance in chronic disease when azathioprine or cyclophosphamide may be used as sparing agents. Rarely, joint arthroplasty may be necessary, although the arthritis can generally be controlled with medication, physiotherapy and splinting.

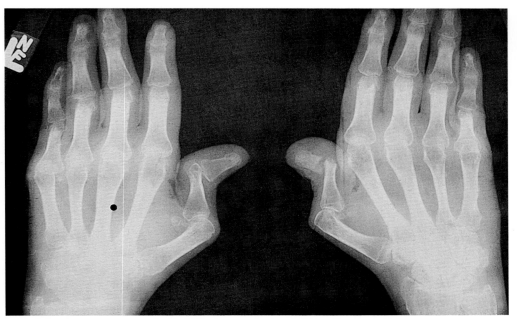

Fig 108.1 **DP hands.** Periarticular osteopenia and multiple subluxations are present. There is little in the way of erosive disease although there is destruction of the base of the thumb terminal phalanx.

109 **Tarsal coalition**

Characteristics
- **Age range:** Probably present at birth but becomes symptomatic in later childhood
- **Gender:** M = F
- **Incidence:** Uncommon
- **Pathology:** Coalition may be bony (synostosis), cartilaginous (synchondrosis) or fibrous (syndesmosis).

Clinical presentation Symptoms arise as ossification progresses and causes hindfoot stress. There may be dorsolateral foot pain and difficulty walking on uneven surfaces with an occasional limp. Examination reveals decreased subtalar movements, tenderness in the region of the sinus tarsi, hindfoot valgus, some loss of the longitudinal arch and, often, peroneal spasm.

Radiology
Description
- The tarsal bones may show bony or fibrous union and radiological interpretation can be difficult
- Lateral view may demonstrate the 'C-sign'

Further imaging
- CT is necessary prior to surgical intervention to define the anatomy

Non-radiological investigations
- None

Management Six weeks of cast immobilization may relieve symptoms for a variable time period, rarely indefinitely. A moulded arch support may help, particularly during activities. Persistent symptoms warrant surgery – either resection of the bar (with muscle or fat interposition), subtalar or triple arthrodesis.

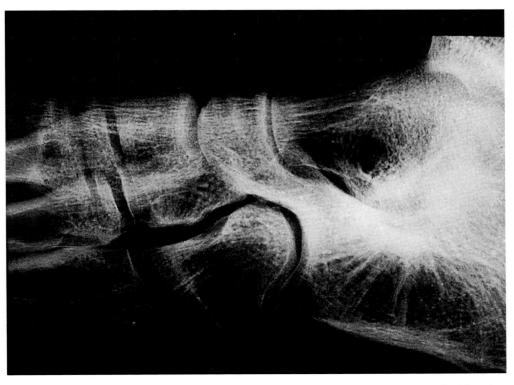

Fig 109.1 **Lateral foot.** There is bony union between the anterior calcaneum and the navicular. Note the abnormal sclerosis at the site of the fusion.

110 **Tendonitis**

Characteristics
- **Age range:** Young adults and middle age
- **Gender:** M = F
- **Incidence:** Common
- **Pathology:** In a true tendonitis there is intratendinous degeneration secondary to atrophy (ageing, microtrauma, vascular compromise, etc.) and histology reveals collagen degeneration, hypocellularity, vascular ingrowth and occasional local necrosis or calcification.

Clinical presentation Pain which increases after exercise and is associated with nodules or a feeling of fullness. It may affect any tendon but commonly the patellar, Achilles tendon and common extensor origin ('tennis elbow').

Radiology
Description
- Plain films may rarely show calcification in diseased tendons

Further imaging
- ☞ US shows the internal architecture of tendons and tendonitis appears as a thickened, hypoechoic tendon
- In severe cases there may be degenerate cysts or calcification
- Peritendonitis may be demonstrated by the presence of peritendonous fluid and thickening of the sheath
- Rotator cuff tendonitis cannot be excluded by US
- MR shows thickening of the tendon with a diffuse increase in signal on T2 weighting

Non-radiological investigations
- None

Management Initially rest and non-steroidal antiinflammatory medication, followed by physiotherapy. If this fails, then local steroid injections can be used although there is a risk of rupture, particularly in the patellar and Achilles tendons. Resistant cases may respond to surgical decompression. In the case of the patellar tendon, this may be achieved arthroscopically.

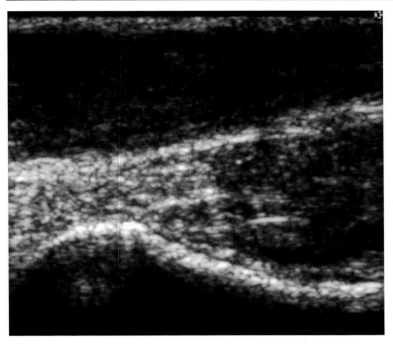

Fig 110.1 **Longitudinal US scan of the Achilles tendon.** There is gross thickening of the tendon with a hypoechoic appearance throughout.

111 Thalassaemia

Characteristics
- **Age range:** May present at any age from birth depending on the type
- **Gender:** M = F
- **Incidence:** Relatively high incidence in those of Mediterranean origin
- **Pathology:** α-Thalassaemia is due to deficiency of α-globin chain synthesis and β-thalassaemia is due to deficiency of β-globin chain synthesis. There are other rare types due to abnormal haemoglobin polypeptide chains δ and δβ. Severity of disease is also determined by homozygote (major) or heterozygote (minor) status.

Clinical presentation
There is anaemia and jaundice with visceral enlargement. Associated abnormalities include endocrine disorders, iron overload and bilirubin stones. The facies is characteristic with a 'rodent' appearance.

Radiology
Description
- 🔑 Changes result from marrow hyperplasia
- Generally thinned cortices with a coarse trabecular pattern
- Widened skull diploic space and thinning of outer table, sparing the occiput
- 'Hair-on-end' appearance
- Small sinuses, ventral displacement of teeth
- Osteoporosis
- Erlenmeyer flask deformity
- Secondary ossification centres appear late
- Epiphyses close early
- Lesions may regress in later life as marrow matures
- Ribs are gradually widened with expanded posterior aspects

Further imaging
- CXR may show cardiomegaly and paravertebral masses
- Abdominal US to look for hepatomegaly and gallstones

Non-radiological investigations
- Full blood count
- Blood film shows raised reticulocytes, normoblasts, target cells and basophilic stippling
- Haemoglobin electrophoresis

Management
Regular blood transfusions and folic acid maintain haemoglobin levels. Iron-chelating agents such as desferrioxamine prevent iron overload. Splenectomy may reduce blood requirements although bone marrow transplantation may be necessary. Endocrine therapy is indicated for delayed puberty. Genetic counselling may be appropriate.

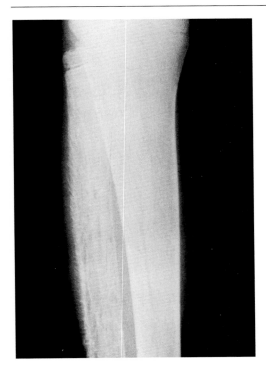

Fig 111.1 **AP lower leg.** Coarse trabeculation is seen, particularly in the fibula, with an associated hair-on-end appearance of the periosteum. There is also some modelling abnormality in the proximal tibia.

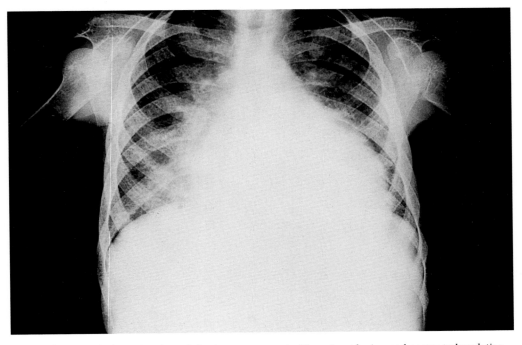

Fig 111.2 **CXR.** The heart is enlarged due to gross anaemia. There is widening and coarse trabeculation of all the bones which is seen best in the ribs.

112 Thyroid acropachy

Characteristics
- **Age range:** Onset is usually 18 months after thyroidectomy for hyperthyroidism
- **Gender:** M = F
- **Incidence:** 1–5% following thyroidectomy
- **Pathology:** The mechanism is unknown but long-acting thyroid stimulator (LATS) has been implicated.

Clinical presentation The patient is characteristically euthyroid or hypothyroid. Presents with clubbing and soft tissue swelling of the fingers, particularly the thumb. It is associated with pretibial myxoedema.

Radiology
Description
- ⚷ Periosteal reaction with a spiculate vertical appearance is seen

- Occurs most often at the metacarpals and metatarsals but sometimes at the distal tibia and fibula

Further imaging
- None

Non-radiological investigations
- Thyroid function tests
- CXR – ☀ the main differential diagnosis is hypertrophic osteoarthropathy

Management It is a self-limiting condition.

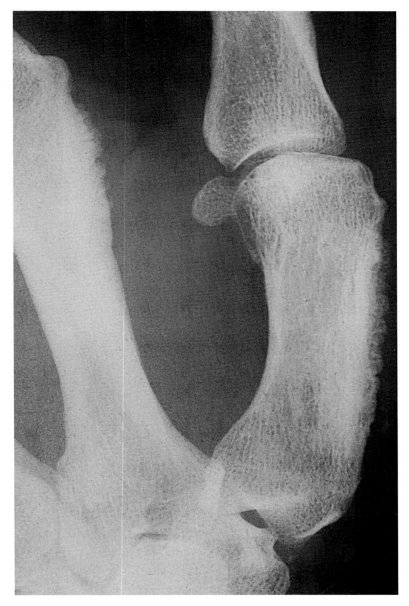

Fig 112.1 **Lateral thumb.** There is mature periosteal reaction along the radial borders of the thumb and index finger metacarpals.

113 **Tuberculosis (TB)**

Characteristics

- **Age range:** Although the initial infection often occurs in childhood it may present at any age
- **Gender:** M = F
- **Incidence:** Becoming more common
- **Pathology:** An acid-alcohol fast bacillus (AAFB) causes a caseating granuloma. The pathogen usually enters the body via the lung or occasionally the gut. Primary infection is usually contained by local lymph nodes and secondary spread occurs later in life, sometimes secondary to immunocompromise, diabetes or debilitation.

Clinical presentation Primary TB is often asymptomatic although there may be fever, cough, sputum or general lethargy. Secondary or postprimary TB is usually symptomatic although symptoms are non-specific, e.g. weight loss, anorexia, night sweats and malaise. Organ-specific symptoms may occur affecting the lungs (haemoptysis, cough, sputum), meningitis, pericarditis, peritonitis or genitourinary tract symptoms. Widespread dissemination may occur via the bloodstream. Bones and joints are affected in 5% of patients, generally vertebral bodies with adjacent collapse and paravertebral abscesses. Larger synovial joints are also affected. Multiple lesions occur in 30%. However, 50% of patients with bone involvement have spinal lesions.

Radiology

Description

- ☛ Soft tissue masses may be seen anterolateral to the vertebral bodies, displacing the paravertebral line or psoas fat stripe
- Disc spaces are reduced with endplate destruction
- Peripherally, lytic lesions are well defined, occasionally mimicking benign neoplastic lesions

- Affected joints show joint space loss and cortical destruction
- Healing occurs with fusion (seen commonly in the hip) and calcification

Further imaging

- Classic changes may be evident on CXR, e.g. upper lobe scarring, calcifications or extensive consolidation and cavitation due to active TB
- MRI of the affected lumbar spine demonstrates high signal in the discs and vertebral bodies with destruction, often at multiple levels
- Psoas abscesses are evident at CT or US
- Imaging-guided abscess drainage
- Imaging-guided aspiration or biopsy

Non-radiological investigations

- Raised ESR
- May be a relative lymphocytosis
- Heaf or Mantoux test is positive
- Synovial fluid has a raised protein content and white cell count
- AAFB identified in 10–20% of aspirates (Ziehl–Nielsen stain) and culture positive in over 50% (Lowenstein–Jensen culture medium) and over 80% positive on histology

Management Rest and splinting of affected joints and then restricted activity for up to a year while changes resolve. Combination therapy is the mainstay of treatment – initially rifampicin, isoniazid, ethambutol and pyrazinamide for 8 weeks and then rifampicin and isoniazid for a further 6 months. Pyridoxine is given throughout. There may be significant side-effects, principally hepatitis, neuropathy and arthralgia. Acute surgical intervention is rarely necessary although 'cold' abscesses may require drainage. In the long term, osteotomies may be needed to correct deformity and destroyed joints may need replacing.

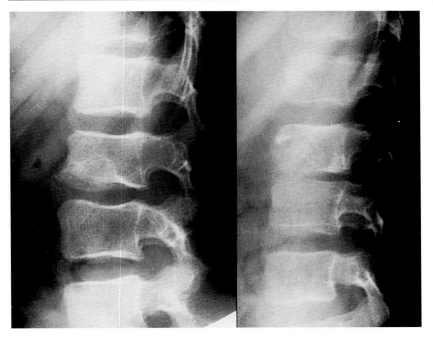

Fig 113.1 **AP spine.** Chronic bony destruction is noted in the vertebral body. There is a mixed pattern of sclerosis and lysis with a relatively well-defined margin.

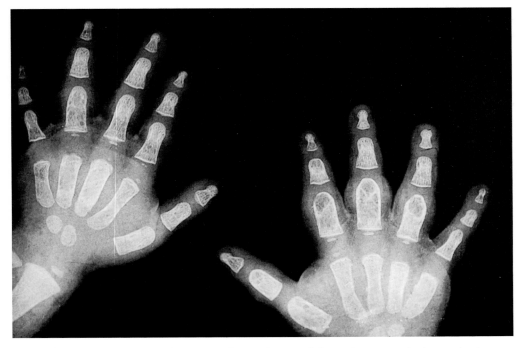

Fig 113.2 **DP hands.** Marked soft tissue swelling and expansile lucencies are seen in the proximal phalanges.